TABLE OF CONTENTS

Top 20 Test Taking Tips

1. Carefully follow all the test registration procedures
2. Know the test directions, duration, topics, question types, how many questions
3. Setup a flexible study schedule at least 3-4 weeks before test day
4. Study during the time of day you are most alert, relaxed, and stress free
5. Maximize your learning style; visual learner use visual study aids, auditory learner use auditory study aids
6. Focus on your weakest knowledge base
7. Find a study partner to review with and help clarify questions
8. Practice, practice, practice
9. Get a good night's sleep; don't try to cram the night before the test
10. Eat a well balanced meal
11. Know the exact physical location of the testing site; drive the route to the site prior to test day
12. Bring a set of ear plugs; the testing center could be noisy
13. Wear comfortable, loose fitting, layered clothing to the testing center; prepare for it to be either cold or hot during the test
14. Bring at least 2 current forms of ID to the testing center
15. Arrive to the test early; be prepared to wait and be patient
16. Eliminate the obviously wrong answer choices, then guess the first remaining choice
17. Pace yourself; don't rush, but keep working and move on if you get stuck
18. Maintain a positive attitude even if the test is going poorly
19. Keep your first answer unless you are positive it is wrong
20. Check your work, don't make a careless mistake

Part I- Vocabulary Review

The Vocabulary test on the exam consists of 30 questions about Word Knowledge.

Word Knowledge

Nearly and Perfect Synonyms

You must determine which of four provided choices has the best similar definition as a certain word. Nearly similar may often be more correct, because the goal is to test your understanding of the nuances, or little differences, between words. A perfect match may not exist, so don't be concerned if your answer choice is not a complete synonym. Focus upon edging closer to the word. Eliminate the words that you know aren't correct first. Then narrow your search. Cross out the words that are the least similar to the main word until you are left with the one that is the most similar.

Prefixes

Take advantage of every clue that the word might include. Prefixes and suffixes can be a huge help. Usually they allow you to determine a basic meaning. Pre- means before, post- means after, pro – is positive, de- is negative. From these prefixes and suffixes, you can get an idea of the general meaning of the word and look for its opposite. Beware though of any traps. Just because con is the opposite of pro, doesn't necessarily mean congress is the opposite of progress! A list of the most common prefixes and suffixes is included in a special report at the end.

Positive vs. Negative

Many words can be easily determined to be a positive word or a negative word. Words such as despicable, gruesome, and bleak are all negative. Words such as ecstatic, praiseworthy, and magnificent are all positive. You will be surprised at how many words can be considered as either positive or negative. Once that is determined, you can quickly eliminate any other words with an opposite meaning and focus on those that have the other characteristic, whether positive or negative.

Word Strength

Part of the challenge is determining the most nearly similar word. This is particularly true when two words seem to be similar. When analyzing a word, determine how strong it is. For example, stupendous and good are both positive words.

However, stupendous is a much stronger positive adjective than good. Also, towering or gigantic are stronger words than tall or large. Search for an answer choice that is similar and also has the same strength. If the main word is weak, look for similar words that are also weak. If the main word is strong, look for similar words that are also strong.

Type and Topic

Another key is what type of word is the main word. If the main word is an adjective describing height, then look for the answer to be an adjective describing height as well. Match both the type and topic of the main word. The type refers the parts of speech, whether the word is an adjective, adverb, or verb. The topic refers to what the definition of the word includes, such as sizes or fashion styles.

Form a Sentence

Many words seem more natural in a sentence. *Specious* reasoning, *irresistible* force, and *uncanny* resemblance are just a few of the word combinations that usually go together. When faced with an uncommon word that you barely understand, try to put the word in a sentence that makes sense. It will help you to understand the word's meaning and make it easier to determine its opposite. Once you have a good descriptive sentence that utilizes the main word properly, plug in the answer choices and see if the sentence still has the same meaning with each answer choice. The answer choice that maintains the meaning of the sentence is correct!

Use Replacements

Using a sentence is a great help because it puts the word into a proper perspective. Since the exam actually gives you a sentence, sometimes you don't always have to create your own (though in many cases the sentence won't be helpful). Read the provided sentence, picking out the main word. Then read the sentence again and again, each time replacing the main word with one of the answer choices. The correct answer should "sound" right and fit.
Example: The desert landscape was desolate. Desolate means
   a.   cheerful
   b.   creepy
   c.   excited
   d.   forlorn

After reading the example sentence, begin replacing "desolate" with each of the answer choices. Does "the desert landscape was cheerful, creepy, excited, or forlorn" sound right? Deserts are typically hot, empty, and rugged environments, probably not cheerful, or excited. While creepy might sound right, that word would certainly be more appropriate for a haunted house. But "the desert landscape was forlorn" has a certain ring to it and would be correct.

Eliminate Similar Choices

If you don't know the word, don't worry. Look at the answer choices and just use them. Remember that three of the answer choices will always be wrong. If you can find a common relationship between any three answer choices, then you know they are wrong. Find the answer choice that does not have a common relationship to the other answer choices and it will be the correct answer.

Example: Laconic most nearly means
- a. wordy
- b. talkative
- c. expressive
- d. quiet

In this example, the first three choices are all similar. Even if you don't know that laconic means the same as quiet, you know that "quiet" must be correct, because the other three choices were all virtually the same. They were all the same, so they must all be wrong. The one that is different must be correct. So, don't worry if you don't know a word. Focus on the answer choices that you do understand and see if you can identify similarities. Even identifying two words that are similar will allow you to eliminate those two answer choices. Because they are similar, they are either both right or both wrong, and since they can't both be right, they must both be wrong.

Example: He worked slowly, moving the leather back and forth until it was ____ .
- a. rough
- b. hard
- c. stiff
- d. pliable

In this example the first three choices are all similar and synonyms. Even without knowing what pliable means, it has to be correct, because you know the other three answer choices mean the same thing.

Adjectives Give it Away

Words mean things and are added to the sentence for a reason. Adjectives in particular may be the clue to determining which answer choice is correct.

Example: The brilliant scientist made several discoveries that were
- a. dull
- b. dazzling

Look at the adjectives first to help determine what makes sense. A "brilliant" or smart scientist would make dazzling, rather than dull discoveries. Without that simple adjective, no answer choice is clear.

Use Logic

Ask yourself questions about each answer choice to see if they are logical.

Example: In the distance, the deep pounding resonance of the drums could be

    a. seen

    b. heard

Would resonating pounding be "seen"? or Would resonating pounding be "heard"?

The Trap of Familiarity

Don't just choose a word because you recognize it. On difficult questions, you may only recognize one or two words. The exam doesn't have "make-believe words" on it, so don't think that just because you only recognize one word means that word must be correct. If you don't recognize four words, then focus on the one that you do recognize. Is it correct? Try your best to determine if it fits the sentence. If it does, that is great, but if it doesn't, eliminate it.

Part I- Mathematics Test Review

The Mathematics Test section of the exam consists of 30 questions. They should not require anything more advanced than 8th grade level math.

Numbers and their Classifications

Numbers are the basic building blocks of mathematics. Specific features of numbers are identified by the following terms:

Integers – The set of whole positive and negative numbers, including zero. Integers do not include fractions ($\frac{1}{3}$), decimals (0.56), or mixed numbers ($7\frac{3}{4}$).

Prime number – A whole number greater than 1 that has only two factors, itself and 1; that is, a number that can be divided evenly only by 1 and itself.

Composite number – A whole number greater than 1 that has more than two different factors; in other words, any whole number that is not a prime number. For example: The composite number 8 has the factors of 1, 2, 4, and 8.

Even number – Any integer that can be divided by 2 without leaving a remainder. For example: 2, 4, 6, 8, and so on.

Odd number – Any integer that cannot be divided evenly by 2. For example: 3, 5, 7, 9, and so on.
Decimal number – a number that uses a decimal point to show the part of the number that is less than one. *Example*: 1.234.

Decimal point – a symbol used to separate the ones place from the tenths place in decimals or dollars from cents in currency.

Decimal place – the position of a number to the right of the decimal point. In the decimal 0.123, the 1 is in the first place to the right of the decimal point, indicating tenths; the 2 is in the second place, indicating hundredths; and the 3 is in the third place, indicating thousandths.

The decimal, or base 10, system is a number system that uses ten different digits (0, 1, 2, 3, 4, 5, 6, 7, 8, 9). An example of a number system that uses something other than ten digits is the binary, or base 2, number system, used by computers, which uses only the numbers 0 and 1. It is thought that the decimal system originated because people had only their 10 fingers for counting.

Rational, irrational, and real numbers can be described as follows:

Rational numbers include all integers, decimals, and fractions. Any terminating or repeating decimal number is a rational number.

Irrational numbers cannot be written as fractions or decimals because the number of decimal places is infinite and there is no recurring pattern of digits within the number. For example, pi (π) begins with 3.141592 and continues without terminating or repeating, so pi is an irrational number.

Real numbers are the set of all rational and irrational numbers.

Operations

There are four basic mathematical operations:

Addition increases the value of one quantity by the value of another quantity.
Example: $2 + 4 = 6; 8 + 9 = 17$. The result is called the sum. With addition, the order does not matter. $4 + 2 = 2 + 4$.

Subtraction is the opposite operation to addition; it decreases the value of one quantity by the value of another quantity.
Example: $6 - 4 = 2; 17 - 8 = 9$. The result is called the difference. Note that with subtraction, the order does matter. $6 - 4 \neq 4 - 6$.

Multiplication can be thought of as repeated addition. One number tells how many times to add the other number to itself.
Example: 3×2 (three times two) $= 2 + 2 + 2 = 6$. With multiplication, the order does not matter. $2 \times 3 = 3 \times 2$ or $3 + 3 = 2 + 2 + 2$.

Division is the opposite operation to multiplication; one number tells us how many parts to divide the other number into.
Example: $20 \div 4 = 5$; if 20 is split into 4 equal parts, each part is 5. With division, the order of the numbers does matter. $20 \div 4 \neq 4 \div 20$.

An exponent is a superscript number placed next to another number at the top right. It indicates how many times the base number is to be multiplied by itself. Exponents provide a shorthand way to write what would be a longer mathematical expression. *Example*: $a^2 = a \times a$; $2^4 = 2 \times 2 \times 2 \times 2$. A number with an exponent of 2 is said to be "squared," while a number with an exponent of 3 is said to be "cubed." The value of a number raised to an exponent is called its power. So, 8^4 is read as "8 to the 4th power," or "8 raised to the power of 4." A negative exponent is the same as the reciprocal of a positive exponent. *Example*: $a^{-2} = \frac{1}{a^2}$.

Parentheses are used to designate which operations should be done first when there are multiple operations.

Example: 4 – (2 + 1) = 1; the parentheses tell us that we must add 2 and 1, and then subtract the sum from 4, rather than subtracting 2 from 4 and then adding 1 (this would give us an answer of 3).

Order of Operations is a set of rules that dictates the order in which we must perform each operation in an expression so that we will evaluate it accurately. If we have an expression that includes multiple different operations, Order of Operations tells us which operations to do first. The most common mnemonic for Order of Operations is PEMDAS, or "Please Excuse My Dear Aunt Sally." PEMDAS stands for Parentheses, Exponents, Multiplication, Division, Addition, Subtraction. It is important to understand that multiplication and division have equal precedence, as do addition and subtraction, so those pairs of operations are simply worked from left to right in order.

> **Review Video: <u>Order of Operations</u>**
> *Visit **mometrix.com/academy** and enter **Code: 259675***

Example: Evaluate the expression $5 + 20 \div 4 \times (2 + 3)^2 - 6$ using the correct order of operations.
P: Perform the operations inside the parentheses, $(2 + 3) = 5$.
E: Simplify the exponents, $(5)^2 = 25$.
The equation now looks like this: $5 + 20 \div 4 \times 25 - 6$.
MD: Perform multiplication and division from left to right, $20 \div 4 = 5$; then $5 \times 25 = 125$.
The equation now looks like this: $5 + 125 - 6$.
AS: Perform addition and subtraction from left to right, $5 + 125 = 130$; then $130 - 6 = 124$.

The laws of exponents are as follows:
1) Any number to the power of 1 is equal to itself: $a^1 = a$.
2) The number 1 raised to any power is equal to 1: $1^n = 1$.
3) Any number raised to the power of 0 is equal to 1: $a^0 = 1$.
4) Add exponents to multiply powers of the same base number: $a^n \times a^m = a^{n+m}$.
5) Subtract exponents to divide powers of the same number; that is $a^n \div a^m = a^{n-m}$.
6) Multiply exponents to raise a power to a power: $(a^n)^m = a^{n \times m}$.
7) If multiplied or divided numbers inside parentheses are collectively raised to a power, this is the same as each individual term being raised to that power: $(a \times b)^n = a^n \times b^n$; $(a \div b)^n = a^n \div b^n$.

Note: Exponents do not have to be integers. Fractional or decimal exponents follow all the rules above as well. *Example*: $5^{\frac{1}{4}} \times 5^{\frac{3}{4}} = 5^{\frac{1}{4}+\frac{3}{4}} = 5^1 = 5$.

A root, such as a square root, is another way of writing a fractional exponent. Instead of using a superscript, roots use the radical symbol ($\sqrt{}$) to indicate the operation. A radical will have a number underneath the bar, and may sometimes have a number in the upper left: $\sqrt[n]{a}$, read as "the nth root of a." The relationship between radical notation and exponent notation can be described by this equation: $\sqrt[n]{a} = a^{\frac{1}{n}}$. The two special cases of n = 2 and n = 3 are called square roots and cube

- 10 -

roots. If there is no number to the upper left, it is understood to be a square root ($n = 2$). Nearly all of the roots you encounter will be square roots. A square root is the same as a number raised to the one-half power. When we say that a is the square root of b ($a = \sqrt{b}$), we mean that a multiplied by itself equals b: ($a \times a = b$).

A perfect square is a number that has an integer for its square root. There are 10 perfect squares from 1 to 100: 1, 4, 9, 16, 25, 36, 49, 64, 81, 100 (the squares of integers 1 through 10).

Scientific notation is a way of writing large numbers in a shorter form. The form $a \times 10^n$ is used in scientific notation, where a is greater than or equal to 1, but less than 10, and n is the number of places the decimal must move to get from the original number to a. *Example*: The number 230,400,000 is cumbersome to write. To write the value in scientific notation, place a decimal point between the first and second numbers, and include all digits through the last non-zero digit ($a = 2.304$). To find the appropriate power of 10, count the number of places the decimal point had to move ($n = 8$). The number is positive if the decimal moved to the left, and negative if it moved to the right. We can then write 230,400,000 as 2.304×10^8.

If we look instead at the number 0.00002304, we have the same value for a, but this time the decimal moved 5 places to the right ($n = -5$). Thus, 0.00002304 can be written as 2.304×10^{-5}. Using this notation makes it simple to compare very large or very small numbers. By comparing exponents, it is easy to see that 3.28×10^4 is smaller than 1.51×10^5, because 4 is less than 5.

Factors and Multiples

Factors are numbers that are multiplied together to obtain a product. For example, in the equation $2 \times 3 = 6$, the numbers 2 and 3 are factors. A prime number has only two factors (1 and itself), but other numbers can have many factors.

A common factor is a number that divides exactly into two or more other numbers. For example, the factors of 12 are 1, 2, 3, 4, 6, and 12, while the factors of 15 are 1, 3, 5, and 15. The common factors of 12 and 15 are 1 and 3.

A prime factor is also a prime number. Therefore, the prime factors of 12 are 2 and 3. For 15, the prime factors are 3 and 5.

The greatest common factor (GCF) is the largest number that is a factor of two or more numbers. For example, the factors of 15 are 1, 3, 5, and 15; the factors of 35 are 1, 5, 7, and 35. Therefore, the greatest common factor of 15 and 35 is 5.

> ➤ **Review Video: <u>Greatest Common Factor</u>**
> *Visit **mometrix.com/academy** and enter **Code: 838699***

The least common multiple (LCM) is the smallest number that is a multiple of two or more numbers. For example, the multiples of 3 include 3, 6, 9, 12, 15, etc.; the multiples of 5 include 5, 10, 15, 20, etc. Therefore, the least common multiple of 3 and 5 is 15.

Fractions, Percentages, and Related Concepts

A fraction is a number that is expressed as one integer written above another integer, with a dividing line between them $\left(\frac{x}{y}\right)$. It represents the quotient of the two numbers "x divided by y." It can also be thought of as x out of y equal parts.

The top number of a fraction is called the numerator, and it represents the number of parts under consideration. The 1 in $\frac{1}{4}$ means that 1 part out of the whole is being considered in the calculation. The bottom number of a fraction is called the denominator, and it represents the total number of equal parts. The 4 in $\frac{1}{4}$ means that the whole consists of 4 equal parts. A fraction cannot have a denominator of zero; this is referred to as "undefined."

Fractions can be manipulated, without changing the value of the fraction, by multiplying or dividing (but not adding or subtracting) both the numerator and denominator by the same number. If you divide both numbers by a common factor, you are reducing or simplifying the fraction. Two fractions that have the same value, but are expressed differently are known as equivalent fractions. For example, $\frac{2}{10}, \frac{3}{15}, \frac{4}{20}$, and $\frac{5}{25}$ are all equivalent fractions. They can also all be reduced or simplified to $\frac{1}{5}$.

When two fractions are manipulated so that they have the same denominator, this is known as finding a common denominator. The number chosen to be that common denominator should be the least common multiple of the two original denominators. *Example:* $\frac{3}{4}$ and $\frac{5}{6}$; the least common multiple of 4 and 6 is 12. Manipulating to achieve the common denominator: $\frac{3}{4} = \frac{9}{12}; \frac{5}{6} = \frac{10}{12}$.

If two fractions have a common denominator, they can be added or subtracted simply by adding or subtracting the two numerators and retaining the same denominator. *Example:* $\frac{1}{2} + \frac{1}{4} = \frac{2}{4} + \frac{1}{4} = \frac{3}{4}$. If the two fractions do not already have the same denominator, one or both of them must be manipulated to achieve a common denominator before they can be added or subtracted.

Two fractions can be multiplied by multiplying the two numerators to find the new numerator and the two denominators to find the new denominator. *Example:* $\frac{1}{3} \times \frac{2}{3} = \frac{1 \times 2}{3 \times 3} = \frac{2}{9}$.

Two fractions can be divided flipping the numerator and denominator of the second fraction and then proceeding as though it were a multiplication. *Example:* $\frac{2}{3} \div \frac{3}{4} = \frac{2}{3} \times \frac{4}{3} = \frac{8}{9}$.

A fraction whose denominator is greater than its numerator is known as a proper fraction, while a fraction whose numerator is greater than its denominator is known as an improper fraction. Proper fractions have values less than one and improper fractions have values greater than one.

A mixed number is a number that contains both an integer and a fraction. Any improper fraction can be rewritten as a mixed number. *Example*: $\frac{8}{3} = \frac{6}{3} + \frac{2}{3} = 2 + \frac{2}{3} = 2\frac{2}{3}$. Similarly, any mixed number can be rewritten as an improper fraction. *Example*: $1\frac{3}{5} = 1 + \frac{3}{5} = \frac{5}{5} + \frac{3}{5} = \frac{8}{5}$.

Percentages can be thought of as fractions that are based on a whole of 100; that is, one whole is equal to 100%. The word percent means "per hundred." Fractions can be expressed as percents by finding equivalent fractions with a denomination of 100. *Example*: $\frac{7}{10} = \frac{70}{100} = 70\%$; $\frac{1}{4} = \frac{25}{100} = 25\%$.

To express a percentage as a fraction, divide the percentage number by 100 and reduce the fraction to its simplest possible terms. *Example*: $60\% = \frac{60}{100} = \frac{3}{5}$; $96\% = \frac{96}{100} = \frac{24}{25}$.

Converting decimals to percentages and percentages to decimals is as simple as moving the decimal point. To convert from a decimal to a percent, move the decimal point two places to the right. To convert from a percent to a decimal, move it two places to the left. *Example*: 0.23 = 23%; 5.34 = 534%; 0.007 = 0.7%; 700% = 7.00; 86% = 0.86; 0.15% = 0.0015.

It may be helpful to remember that the percentage number will always be larger than the equivalent decimal number.

A percentage problem can be presented three main ways: (1) Find what percentage of some number another number is. *Example*: What percentage of 40 is 8? (2) Find what number is some percentage of a given number. *Example*: What number is 20% of 40? (3) Find what number another number is a given percentage of. *Example*: What number is 8 20% of? The three components in all of these cases are the same: a whole (W), a part (P), and a percentage (%). These are related by the equation: $P = W \times \%$. This is the form of the equation you would use to solve problems of type (2). To solve types (1) and (3), you would use these two forms: $\% = \frac{P}{W}$ and $W = \frac{P}{\%}$.

The thing that frequently makes percentage problems difficult is that they are most often also word problems, so a large part of solving them is figuring out which quantities are what. *Example*: In a school cafeteria, 7 students choose pizza, 9 choose hamburgers, and 4 choose tacos. Find the percentage that chooses tacos. To find the whole, you must first add all of the parts: 7 + 9 + 4 = 20. The percentage can then be found by dividing the part by the whole ($\% = \frac{P}{W}$): $\frac{4}{20} = \frac{20}{100} = 20\%$.

A ratio is a comparison of two quantities in a particular order. *Example*: If there are 14 computers in a lab, and the class has 20 students, there is a student to computer ratio of 20 to 14, commonly written as 20:14. Ratios are normally reduced to their smallest whole number representation, so 20:14 would be reduced to 10:7 by dividing both sides by 2.

A proportion is a relationship between two quantities that dictates how one changes when the other changes. A direct proportion describes a relationship in which a quantity increases by a set amount for every increase in the other quantity, or decreases by that same amount for every decrease in the other quantity.

Example: Assuming a constant driving speed, the time required for a car trip increases as the distance of the trip increases. The distance to be traveled and the time required to travel are directly proportional.

Inverse proportion is a relationship in which an increase in one quantity is accompanied by a decrease in the other, or vice versa.

Example: the time required for a car trip decreases as the speed increases, and increases as the speed decreases, so the time required is inversely proportional to the speed of the car.

Part I – Form Relationship Test

The Part I Form Relationship Test requires you to visualize differences in object and manipulate things mentally.

Work Fast

The problems can be real brain teasers, because for most questions you would be able to figure out the correct answer if you had an infinite amount of time. That's why on this section more than any other you have to be conscious of time.

Rule Busters

Each problem provides you with some known information in the form of a relationship between two shapes. Look at the relationship given and decide what obvious characteristics the correct answer needs to have. These are the rules that you have to work with. Rule busters are answer choices that immediately clash with a rule and can be quickly ruled out.
Example: The given pair of shapes are both circles. The first shape in the pair that you must complete is a square, so your choice must be a square.

This is a rule. Therefore, any answer choice that is not a square is a rule buster, and is wrong! Quickly scan through the list of answer choices and eliminate all of those that are not squares.

Identify the Odd Shape

Find the most unusual feature that the correct answer needs to have, and then check the answer choices for a shape containing that feature. Don't waste time on the common features, but find the unusual feature and spend your time looking only among the answer choices that have it.

Process of Elimination

If you can't figure out which one is best, figure out which ones are worst. If you can safely eliminate certain answer choices, then you improve your chances at a guess and with the tight time restrictions you face, guessing will be an important part of your strategy on this particular test section.

Identify the Differences

What is different between the answer choices given? If all the answer choices are the same shape, don't waste time trying to figure out what shape the correct answer should be. Focus on the features that are different and then you can narrow your answer choice down to the correct answer.

Tough Questions

If you are stumped on a problem or it appears too hard or too difficult, don't waste time. Move on! Remember though, if you can quickly check for obvious "rule busters" your chances of guessing correctly are greatly improved. Before you completely give up, at least check for the easy rule busters, which should knock out a couple of possible answers. Eliminate what you can and then guess at the remainder before moving on.

Answer Selection

Eliminate choices as soon as you realize they are wrong. But be careful! Make sure you consider all of the possible answer choices. Just because one appears right, doesn't mean that the next one won't be even better! Don't worry if you are stuck between two that seem right and can't figure out which is the one. By eliminating the other choices your odds of guessing right are now 50/50 if you have it down to two. Rather than wasting too much time, play the odds. You are guessing, but guessing wisely, because you've been able to knock out some of the answer choices that you know are wrong. If you are eliminating choices and realize that the answer choice you are left with is also obviously wrong, don't panic. Start over and consider each choice again. There may easily be something that you missed the first time and will realize on the second pass.

The best way to pick an answer choice is to eliminate all of those that are wrong, until only one is left and confirm that is the correct answer and meets all of the established rules. Sometimes though, an answer choice may immediately look right. Be careful! Take a second to make sure that the other choices are not equally obvious. Don't make a hasty mistake. There are only two times that you should move on before checking other answers. First is when you are positive that the answer choice you have selected satisfies all of the rules. Second is when time is almost out and you have to make a quick guess!

Final Notes

Some problems may require that you understand a complex relationship between two shapes. Always use your time efficiently. Don't panic, stay focused. Work systematically. View the answer choices carefully. Eliminate the ones that are immediately wrong. Keep narrowing the search until you are either left with the answer or must guess at the answer from a more selective group of choices. This strategy will maximize your score on this section.

Part II – Spelling Test

It is extremely difficult to teach someone how to be a good speller, if they have been a bad speller all their life. Becoming a good speller takes lots of time. That is why we have decided to create a link review for this section of this test. Use the links listed below to work on your spelling to succeed on the test.

http://www.aaaspell.com/spelling/8

http://eslus.com/LESSONS/SPELL/SPELL.HTM

http://www.esl-lounge.com/quiz-spelling.shtml

Part III - Reading Comprehension

In order to be an effective reader, one must pay attention to the author's **position** and purpose. Even those texts that seem objective and impartial, like textbooks, have some sort of position and bias. Readers need to take these positions into account when considering the author's message. When an author uses emotional language or clearly favors one side of an argument, his position is clear. However, the author's position may be evident not only in what he writes, but in what he doesn't write. For this reason, it is sometimes necessary to review some other texts on the same topic in order to develop a view of the author's position. If this is not possible, then it may be useful to acquire a little background personal information about the author. When the only source of information is the text, however, the reader should look for language and argumentation that seems to indicate a particular stance on the subject.

Identifying the **purpose** of an author is usually easier than identifying her position. In most cases, the author has no interest in hiding his or her purpose. A text that is meant to entertain, for instance, should be obviously written to please the reader. Most narratives, or stories, are written to entertain, though they may also inform or persuade. Informative texts are easy to identify as well. The most difficult purpose of a text to identify is persuasion, because the author has an interest in making this purpose hard to detect. When a person knows that the author is trying to convince him, he is automatically more wary and skeptical of the argument. For this reason persuasive texts often try to establish an entertaining tone, hoping to amuse the reader into agreement, or an informative tone, hoping to create an appearance of authority and objectivity.

> ➢ **Review Video: <u>Purpose of an Author</u>**
> *Visit **mometrix.com/academy** and enter **Code: 497555**

An author's purpose is often evident in the organization of the text. For instance, if the text has headings and subheadings, if key terms are in bold, and if the author makes his main idea clear from the beginning, then the likely purpose of the text is to inform. If the author begins by making a claim and then makes various arguments to support that claim, the purpose is probably to persuade. If the author is telling a story, or is more interested in holding the attention of the reader than in making a particular point or delivering information, then his purpose is most likely to entertain. As a reader, it is best to judge an author on how well he accomplishes his purpose. In other words, it is not entirely fair to complain that a textbook is boring: if the text is clear and easy to understand, then the author has done his job. Similarly, a storyteller should not be judged too harshly for getting some facts wrong, so long as he is able to give pleasure to the reader.

The author's purpose for writing will affect his writing style and the response of the reader. In a **persuasive essay**, the author is attempting to change the reader's mind or convince him of something he did not believe previously. There are several identifying characteristics of persuasive writing. One is opinion presented as fact. When an author attempts to persuade the reader, he often presents his or her opinions as if they were fact. A reader must be on guard for statements that sound factual but which cannot be subjected to research, observation, or experiment. Another characteristic of persuasive writing is emotional language. An author will often try to play on the reader's emotion by appealing to his sympathy or sense of morality. When an author uses colorful or evocative language with the intent of arousing the reader's passions, it is likely that he is attempting to persuade. Finally, in many cases a persuasive text will give an unfair explanation of opposing positions, if these positions are mentioned at all.

➢ **Review Video: Persuasive Essay**
Visit ***mometrix.com/academy*** *and enter* *Code:* **621428**

An **informative text** is written to educate and enlighten the reader. Informative texts are almost always nonfiction, and are rarely structured as a story. The intention of an informative text is to deliver information in the most comprehensible way possible, so the structure of the text is likely to be very clear. In an informative text, the thesis statement is often in the first sentence. The author may use some colorful language, but is likely to put more emphasis on clarity and precision. Informative essays do not typically appeal to the emotions. They often contain facts and figures, and rarely include the opinion of the author. Sometimes a persuasive essay can resemble an informative essay, especially if the author maintains an even tone and presents his or her views as if they were established fact.

➢ **Review Video: Informative Text**
Visit ***mometrix.com/academy*** *and enter* *Code:* **924964**

The success or failure of an author's intent to **entertain** is determined by those who read the author's work. Entertaining texts may be either fiction or nonfiction, and they may describe real or imagined people, places, and events. Entertaining texts are often narratives, or stories. A text that is written to entertain is likely to contain colorful language that engages the imagination and the emotions. Such writing often features a great deal of figurative language, which typically enlivens its subject matter with images and analogies. Though an entertaining text is not usually written to persuade or inform, it may accomplish both of these tasks. An entertaining text may appeal to the reader's emotions and cause him or her to think differently about a particular subject. In any case, entertaining texts tend to showcase the personality of the author more so than do other types of writing.

When an author intends to **express feelings,** she may use colorful and evocative language. An author may write emotionally for any number of reasons. Sometimes, the author will do so because she is describing a personal situation of great pain or happiness. Sometimes an author is attempting to persuade the reader, and so will use emotion to stir up the passions. It can be easy to identify this kind of expression when the writer uses phrases like *I felt* and *I sense*.

➢ **Review Video: Express Feelings**
Visit ***mometrix.com/academy*** *and enter* *Code:* **759390**

However, sometimes the author will simply describe feelings without introducing them. As a reader, it is important to recognize when an author is expressing emotion, and not to become overwhelmed by sympathy or passion. A reader should maintain some detachment so that he or she can still evaluate the strength of the author's argument or the quality of the writing.

In a sense, almost all writing is descriptive, insofar as it seeks to describe events, ideas, or people to the reader. Some texts, however, are primarily concerned with **description**. A descriptive text focuses on a particular subject, and attempts to depict it in a way that will be clear to the reader. Descriptive texts contain many adjectives and adverbs, words that give shades of meaning and create a more detailed mental picture for the reader. A descriptive text fails when it is unclear or vague to the reader. On the other hand, however, a descriptive text that compiles too much detail can be boring and overwhelming to the reader. A descriptive text will certainly be informative, and it may be persuasive and entertaining as well. Descriptive writing is a challenge for the author, but when it is done well, it can be fun to read.

Writing Devices

Authors will use different stylistic and writing devices to make their meaning more clearly understood. One of those devices is comparison and contrast. When an author describes the ways in which two things are alike, he or she is **comparing** them. When the author describes the ways in which two things are different, he or she is **contrasting** them. The "compare and contrast" essay is one of the most common forms in nonfiction. It is often signaled with certain words: a comparison may be indicated with such words as *both*, *same*, *like*, *too*, and *as well*; while a contrast may be indicated by words like *but*, *however*, *on the other hand*, *instead*, and *yet*. Of course, comparisons and contrasts may be implicit without using any such signaling language. A single sentence may both compare and contrast. Consider the sentence *Brian and Sheila love ice cream, but Brian prefers vanilla and Sheila prefers strawberry*. In one sentence, the author has described both a similarity (love of ice cream) and a difference (favorite flavor).

> ➤ **Review Video: <u>Compare and Contrast</u>**
> *Visit **mometrix.com/academy** and enter **Code: 798319***

One of the most common text structures is **cause and effect**. A cause is an act or event that makes something happen, and an effect is the thing that happens as a result of that cause. A cause-and-effect relationship is not always explicit, but there are some words in English that signal causality, such as *since*, *because*, and *as a result*. As an example, consider the sentence *Because the sky was clear, Ron did not bring an umbrella*. The cause is the clear sky, and the effect is that Ron did not bring an umbrella. However, sometimes the cause-and-effect relationship will not be clearly noted. For instance, the sentence *He was late and missed the meeting* does not contain any signaling words, but it still contains a cause (he was late) and an effect (he missed the meeting). It is possible for a single cause to have multiple effects, or for a single effect to have multiple causes. Also, an effect can in turn be the cause of another effect, in what is known as a cause-and-effect chain.

Authors often use analogies to add meaning to the text. An **analogy** is a comparison of two things. The words in the analogy are connected by a certain, often undetermined relationship. Look at this

- 20 -

analogy: moo is to cow as quack is to duck. This analogy compares the sound that a cow makes with the sound that a duck makes. Even if the word 'quack' was not given, one could figure out it is the correct word to complete the analogy based on the relationship between the words 'moo' and 'cow'. Some common relationships for analogies include synonyms, antonyms, part to whole, definition, and actor to action.

Another element that impacts a text is the author's point of view. The **point of view** of a text is the perspective from which it is told. The author will always have a point of view about a story before he draws up a plot line. The author will know what events they want to take place, how they want the characters to interact, and how the story will resolve. An author will also have an opinion on the topic, or series of events, which is presented in the story, based on their own prior experience and beliefs.

> **Review Video: <u>Point of View</u>**
> *Visit **mometrix.com/academy** and enter **Code: 383336***

The two main points of view that authors use are first person and third person. If the narrator of the story is also the main character, or *protagonist*, the text is written in first-person point of view. In first person, the author writes with the word *I*. Third-person point of view is probably the most common point of view that authors use. Using third person, authors refer to each character using the words *he* or *she*. In third-person omniscient, the narrator is not a character in the story and tells the story of all of the characters at the same time.

A good writer will use **transitional words** and phrases to guide the reader through the text. You are no doubt familiar with the common transitions, though you may never have considered how they operate. Some transitional phrases (*after, before, during, in the middle of*) give information about time. Some indicate that an example is about to be given (*for example, in fact, for instance*). Writers use them to compare (*also, likewise*) and contrast (*however, but, yet*). Transitional words and phrases can suggest addition (*and, also, furthermore, moreover*) and logical relationships (*if, then, therefore, as a result, since*). Finally, transitional words and phrases can demarcate the steps in a process (*first, second, last*). You should incorporate transitional words and phrases where they will orient your reader and illuminate the structure of your composition.

> **Review Video: <u>Transitional Words and Phrases</u>**
> *Visit **mometrix.com/academy** and enter **Code: 197796***

Types of Passages

A **narrative** passage is a story. Narratives can be fiction or nonfiction. However, there are a few elements that a text must have in order to be classified as a narrative. To begin with, the text must have a plot. That is, it must describe a series of events. If it is a good narrative, these events will be interesting and emotionally engaging to the reader. A narrative also has characters. These could be people, animals, or even inanimate objects, so long as they participate in the plot. A narrative passage often contains figurative language, which is meant to stimulate the imagination of the reader by making comparisons and observations. A metaphor, which is a description of one thing in terms of another, is a common piece of figurative language. *The moon was a frosty snowball* is an example of a metaphor: it is obviously untrue in the literal sense, but it suggests a certain mood for the reader. Narratives often proceed in a clear sequence, but they do not need to do so.

> ➤ **Review Video: <u>Narratives</u>**
> *Visit **mometrix.com/academy** and enter **Code: 280100***

An **expository** passage aims to inform and enlighten the reader. It is nonfiction and usually centers around a simple, easily defined topic. Since the goal of exposition is to teach, such a passage should be as clear as possible. It is common for an expository passage to contain helpful organizing words, like *first, next, for example,* and *therefore*. These words keep the reader oriented in the text. Although expository passages do not need to feature colorful language and artful writing, they are often more effective when they do. For a reader, the challenge of expository passages is to maintain steady attention. Expository passages are not always about subjects in which a reader will naturally be interested, and the writer is often more concerned with clarity and comprehensibility than with engaging the reader. For this reason, many expository passages are dull. Making notes is a good way to maintain focus when reading an expository passage.

> ➤ **Review Video: <u>Expository Passages</u>**
> *Visit **mometrix.com/academy** and enter **Code: 256515***

A **technical** passage is written to describe a complex object or process. Technical writing is common in medical and technological fields, in which complicated mathematical, scientific, and engineering ideas need to be explained simply and clearly. To ease comprehension, a technical passage usually proceeds in a very logical order. Technical passages often have clear headings and subheadings, which are used to keep the reader oriented in the text. It is also common for these passages to break sections up with numbers or letters. Many technical passages look more like an outline than a piece of prose. The amount of jargon or difficult vocabulary will vary in a technical passage depending on the intended audience. As much as possible, technical passages try to avoid language that the reader will have to research in order to understand the message. Of course, it is not always possible to avoid jargon.

A **persuasive** passage is meant to change the reader's mind or lead her into agreement with the author. The persuasive intent may be obvious, or it may be quite difficult to discern. In some cases, a persuasive passage will be indistinguishable from an informative passage: it will make an assertion and offer supporting details. However, a persuasive passage is more likely to make claims based on opinion and to appeal to the reader's emotions.

Persuasive passages may not describe alternate positions and, when they do, they often display significant bias. It may be clear that a persuasive passage is giving the author's viewpoint, or the passage may adopt a seemingly objective tone. A persuasive passage is successful if it can make a convincing argument and win the trust of the reader.

A persuasive essay will likely focus on one central argument, but it may make many smaller claims along the way. These are subordinate arguments with which the reader must agree if he or she is going to agree with the central argument. The central argument will only be as strong as the subordinate claims. These claims should be rooted in fact and observation, rather than subjective judgment. The best persuasive essays provide enough supporting detail to justify claims without overwhelming the reader. Remember that a fact must be susceptible to independent verification: that is, it must be something the reader could confirm. Also, statistics are only effective when they take into account possible objections. For instance, a statistic on the number of foreclosed houses would only be useful if it was taken over a defined interval and in a defined area. Most readers are wary of statistics, because they are so often misleading. If possible, a persuasive essay should always include references so that the reader can obtain more information. Of course, this means that the writer's accuracy and fairness may be judged by the inquiring reader.

Opinions are formed by emotion as well as reason, and persuasive writers often appeal to the feelings of the reader. Although readers should always be skeptical of this technique, it is often used in a proper and ethical manner. For instance, there are many subjects that have an obvious emotional component, and therefore cannot be completely treated without an appeal to the emotions. Consider an article on drunk driving: it makes sense to include some specific examples that will alarm or sadden the reader. After all, drunk driving often has serious and tragic consequences. Emotional appeals are not appropriate, however, when they attempt to mislead the reader. For instance, in political advertisements it is common to emphasize the patriotism of the preferred candidate, because this will encourage the audience to link their own positive feelings about the country with their opinion of the candidate. However, these ads often imply that the other candidate is unpatriotic, which in most cases is far from the truth. Another common and improper emotional appeal is the use of loaded language, as for instance referring to an avidly religious person as a "fanatic" or a passionate environmentalist as a "tree hugger." These terms introduce an emotional component that detracts from the argument.

> **Review Video: <u>Persuasive Techniques</u>**
> *Visit **mometrix.com/academy** and enter **Code: 577997***

Responding to Literature

When reading good literature, the reader is moved to engage actively in the text. One part of being an active reader involves making predictions. A **prediction** is a guess about what will happen next. Readers are constantly making predictions based on what they have read and what they already know. Consider the following sentence: *Staring at the computer screen in shock, Kim blindly reached over for the brimming glass of water on the shelf to her side.* The sentence suggests that Kim is agitated and that she is not looking at the glass she is going to pick up, so a reader might predict that she is going to knock the glass over.

> **Review Video: <u>Prediction</u>**
> *Visit **mometrix.com/academy** and enter **Code: 437248***

Of course, not every prediction will be accurate: perhaps Kim will pick the glass up cleanly. Nevertheless, the author has certainly created the expectation that the water might be spilled. Predictions are always subject to revision as the reader acquires more information.

Test-taking tip: To respond to questions requiring future predictions, the student's answers should be based on evidence of past or present behavior.

Readers are often required to understand text that claims and suggests ideas without stating them directly. An **inference** is a piece of information that is implied but not written outright by the author. For instance, consider the following sentence: *Mark made more money that week than he had in the previous year*. From this sentence, the reader can infer that Mark either has not made much money in the previous year or made a great deal of money that week. Often, a reader can use information he or she already knows to make inferences. Take as an example the sentence *When his coffee arrived, he looked around the table for the silver cup*. Many people know that cream is typically served in a silver cup, so using their own base of knowledge they can infer that the subject of this sentence takes his coffee with cream. Making inferences requires concentration, attention, and practice.

> **Review Video: Inference**
> *Visit mometrix.com/academy* and enter *Code: 379203*

Test-taking tip: While being tested on his ability to make correct inferences, the student must look for contextual clues. An answer can be *true* but not *correct*. The contextual clues will help you find the answer that is the best answer out of the given choices. Understand the context in which a phrase is stated. When asked for the implied meaning of a statement made in the passage, the student should immediately locate the statement and read the context in which it was made. Also, look for an answer choice that has a similar phrase to the statement in question.

A reader must be able to identify a text's **sequence**, or the order in which things happen. Often, and especially when the sequence is very important to the author, it is indicated with signal words like *first*, *then*, *next*, and *last*. However, sometimes a sequence is merely implied and must be noted by the reader. Consider the sentence *He walked in the front door and switched on the hall lamp*. Clearly, the man did not turn the lamp on before he walked in the door, so the implied sequence is that he first walked in the door and then turned on the lamp. Texts do not always proceed in an orderly sequence from first to last: sometimes, they begin at the end and then start over at the beginning. As a reader, it can be useful to make brief notes to clarify the sequence.

> **Review Video: Sequence**
> *Visit mometrix.com/academy* and enter *Code: 489027*

In addition to inferring and predicting things about the text, the reader must often **draw conclusions** about the information he has read. When asked for a *conclusion* that may be drawn, look for critical "hedge" phrases, such as *likely*, *may*, *can*, *will often*, among many others. When you are being tested on this knowledge, remember that question writers insert these hedge phrases to cover every possibility. Often an answer will be wrong simply because it leaves no room for exception. Extreme positive or negative answers (such as always, never, etc.) are usually not correct. The reader should not use any outside knowledge that is not gathered from the reading passage to answer the related questions. Correct answers can be derived straight from the reading passage.

Testing Tips

Skimming

Your first task when you begin reading is to answer the question "What is the topic of the selection?" This can best be answered by quickly skimming the passage for the general idea, stopping to read only the first sentence of each paragraph. A paragraph's first sentence is usually the main topic sentence, and it gives you a summary of the content of the paragraph.

Once you've skimmed the passage, stopping to read only the first sentences, you will have a general idea about what it is about, as well as what is the expected topic in each paragraph.

Each question will contain clues as to where to find the answer in the passage. Do not just randomly search through the passage for the correct answer to each question. Search scientifically. Find key word(s) or ideas in the question that are going to either contain or be near the correct answer. These are typically nouns, verbs, numbers, or phrases in the question that will probably be duplicated in the passage. Once you have identified those key word(s) or idea, skim the passage quickly to find where those key word(s) or idea appears. The correct answer choice will be nearby. *Example*: What caused Martin to suddenly return to Paris?

The key word is Paris. Skim the passage quickly to find where this word appears. The answer will be close by that word.

However, sometimes key words in the question are not repeated in the passage. In those cases, search for the general idea of the question.
Example: Which of the following was the psychological impact of the author's childhood upon the remainder of his life?

Key words are "childhood" or "psychology". While searching for those words, be alert for other words or phrases that have similar meaning, such as "emotional effect" or "mentally" which could be used in the passage, rather than the exact word "psychology".

Numbers or years can be particularly good key words to skim for, as they stand out from the rest of the text.
Example: Which of the following best describes the influence of Monet's work in the 20th century? 20th contains numbers and will easily stand out from the rest of the text. Use 20th as the key word to skim for in the passage.

Other good key word(s) may be in quotation marks. These identify a word or phrase that is copied directly from the passage. In those cases, the word(s) in quotation marks are exactly duplicated in the passage.

Example: In her college years, what was meant by Margaret's "drive for excellence"?

"Drive for excellence" is a direct quote from the passage and should be easy to find.

Once you've quickly found the correct section of the passage to find the answer, focus upon the answer choices. Sometimes a choice will repeat word for word a portion of the passage near the answer. However, beware of such duplication – it may be a trap! More than likely, the correct choice will paraphrase or summarize the related portion of the passage, rather than being exactly the same wording.

For the answers that you think are correct, read them carefully and make sure that they answer the question. An answer can be factually correct, but it MUST answer the question asked. Additionally, two answers can both be seemingly correct, so be sure to read all of the answer choices, and make sure that you get the one that BEST answers the question.

Some questions will not have a key word.
Example: Which of the following would the author of this passage likely agree with?

In these cases, look for key words in the answer choices. Then skim the passage to find where the answer choice occurs. By skimming to find where to look, you can minimize the time required.

Sometimes it may be difficult to identify a good key word in the question to skim for in the passage. In those cases, look for a key word in one of the answer choices to skim for. Often the answer choices can all be found in the same paragraph, which can quickly narrow your search.

Paragraph Focus

Focus upon the first sentence of each paragraph, which is the most important. The main topic of the paragraph is usually there.

Once you've read the first sentence in the paragraph, you have a general idea about what each paragraph will be about. As you read the questions, try to determine which paragraph will have the answer. Paragraphs have a concise topic. The answer should either obviously be there or obviously not. It will save time if you can jump straight to the paragraph, so try to remember what you learned from the first sentences.
Example: The first paragraph is about poets; the second is about poetry. If a question asks about poetry, where will the answer be? *The second paragraph.*

The main idea of a passage is typically spread across all or most of its paragraphs. Whereas the main idea of a paragraph may be completely different than the main idea of the very next paragraph, a main idea for a passage affects all of the paragraphs in one form or another. *Example*: What is the main idea of the passage?

For each answer choice, try to see how many paragraphs are related. It can help to count how many sentences are affected by each choice, but it is best to see how many paragraphs are affected by the choice. Typically the answer choices will include incorrect choices that are main ideas of individual paragraphs, but not the entire passage. That is why it is crucial to choose ideas that are supported by the most paragraphs possible.

Eliminate Choices

Some choices can quickly be eliminated. "Andy Warhol lived there." Is Andy Warhol even mentioned in the article? If not, quickly eliminate it.

When trying to answer a question such as "the passage indicates all of the following EXCEPT" quickly skim the paragraph searching for references to each choice. If the reference exists, scratch it off as a choice. Similar choices may be crossed off simultaneously if they are close enough.

In choices that ask you to choose "which answer choice does NOT describe?" or "all of the following answer choices are identifiable characteristics, EXCEPT which?" look for answers that are similarly worded. Since only one answer can be correct, if there are two answers that appear to mean the same thing, they must BOTH be incorrect, and can be eliminated.
Example:
  a. changing values and attitudes
  b. a large population of mobile or uprooted people

These answer choices are similar; they both describe a fluid culture. Because of their similarity, they can be linked together. Since the answer can have only one choice, they can also be eliminated together.

Contextual Clues

Look for contextual clues. An answer can be right but not correct. The contextual clues will help you find the answer that is most right and is correct. Understand the context in which a phrase is stated.

When asked for the implied meaning of a statement made in the passage, immediately go find the statement and read the context it was made in. Also, look for an answer choice that has a similar phrase to the statement in question.
Example: In the passage, what is implied by the phrase "Churches have become more or less part of the furniture"?

Find an answer choice that is similar or describes the phrase "part of the furniture" as that is the key phrase in the question. "Part of the furniture" is a saying that means something is fixed, immovable, or set in their ways. Those are all similar ways of saying "part of the furniture." As such, the correct answer choice will probably include a similar rewording of the expression.
Example: Why was John described as "morally desperate"?

The answer will probably have some sort of definition of morals in it. "Morals" refers to a code of right and wrong behavior, so the correct answer choice will likely have words that mean something like that.

Fact/Opinion

When asked about which statement is a fact or opinion, remember that answer choices that are facts will typically have no ambiguous words. For example, how long is a long time? What defines an ordinary person? These ambiguous words of "long" and "ordinary" should not be in a factual statement. However, if all of the choices have ambiguous words, go to the context of the passage. Often a factual statement may be set out as a research finding.
Example: "The scientist found that the eye reacts quickly to change in light."

Opinions may be set out in the context of words like thought, believed, understood, or wished.
Example: "He thought the Yankees should win the World Series."

Opposites

When two answer choices are direct opposites, one of them is usually correct. The paragraph will often contain established relationships (when this goes up, that goes down). The question may ask you to draw conclusions for this and will give two similar answer choices that are opposites.
Example:
   a.   a decrease in housing starts
   b.   an increase in housing starts

Make Predictions

As you read and understand the passage and then the question, try to guess what the answer will be. Remember that three of the four answer choices are wrong, and once you being reading them, your mind will immediately become cluttered with answer choices designed to throw you off. Your mind is typically the most focused immediately after you have read the passage and question and digested its contents. If you can, try to predict what the correct answer will be. You may be surprised at what you can predict.

Quickly scan the choices and see if your prediction is in the listed answer choices. If it is, then you can be quite confident that you have the right answer. It still won't hurt to check the other answer choices, but most of the time, you've got it!

Answer the Question

It may seem obvious to only pick answer choices that answer the question, but the exam can contain some excellent answer choices that are wrong. Don't pick an answer just because it sounds right, or you believe it to be true. It MUST answer the question. Once you've made your selection, always go back and check it against the question and make sure that you didn't misread the question, and the answer choice does answer the question posed.

Benchmark

After you read the first answer choice, decide if you think it sounds correct or not. If it doesn't, move on to the next answer choice. If it does, make a mental note about that choice. This doesn't mean that you've definitely selected it as your answer choice, it just means that it's the best you've seen thus far. Go ahead and read the next choice. If the next choice is worse than the one you've already selected, keep going to the next answer choice. If the next choice is better than the choice you've already selected, then make a mental note about that answer choice.

As you read through the list, you are mentally noting the choice you think is right. That is your new standard. Every other answer choice must be benchmarked against that standard. That choice is correct until proven otherwise by another answer choice beating it out. Once you've decided that no other answer choice seems as good, do one final check to ensure that it answers the question posed.

New Information

Correct answers will usually contain the information listed in the paragraph and question. Rarely will completely new information be inserted into a correct answer choice. Occasionally the new information may be related in a manner that the exam is asking for you to interpret, but seldom. *Example*: The argument above is dependent upon which of the following assumptions?
   a. Charles's Law was used

If Charles's Law is not mentioned at all in the referenced paragraph and argument, then it is unlikely that this choice is correct. All of the information needed to answer the question is provided for you, and so you should not have to make guesses that are unsupported or choose answer choices that have unknown information that cannot be reasoned.

Valid Information

Don't discount any of the information provided in the passage, particularly shorter ones. Every piece of information may be necessary to determine the correct answer. None of the information in the paragraph is there to throw you off (while the answer choices will certainly have information to throw you off). If two seemingly unrelated topics are discussed, don't ignore either. You can be confident there is a relationship, or it wouldn't be included in the paragraph, and you are probably going to have to determine what is that relationship for the answer.

Time Management

In technical passages, do not get lost on the technical terms. Skip them and move on. You want a general understanding of what is going on, not a mastery of the passage.

When you encounter material in the selection that seems difficult to understand, it often may not be necessary and can be skipped. Only spend time trying to understand it if it is going to be relevant for a question. Understand difficult phrases only as a last resort.

Answer general questions before detail questions. A reader with a good understanding of the whole passage can often answer general questions without rereading a word. Get the easier questions out of the way before tackling the more time consuming ones.

Identify each question by type. Usually the wording of a question will tell you whether you can find the answer by referring directly to the passage or by using your reasoning powers. You alone know which question types you customarily handle with ease and which give you trouble and will require more time. Save the difficult questions for last.

Final Warnings

Word Usage Questions

When asked how a word is used in the passage, don't use your existing knowledge of the word. The question is being asked precisely because there is some strange or unusual usage of the word in the passage. Go to the passage and use contextual clues to determine the answer. Don't simply use the popular definition you already know.

Switchback Words

Stay alert for "switchbacks". These are the words and phrases frequently used to alert you to shifts in thought. The most common switchback word is "but". Others include although, however, nevertheless, on the other hand, even though, while, in spite of, despite, regardless of.

Avoid "Fact Traps"

Once you know which paragraph the answer will be in, focus on that paragraph. However, don't get distracted by a choice that is factually true about the paragraph. Your search is for the answer that answers the question, which may be about a tiny aspect in the paragraph. Stay focused and don't fall for an answer that describes the larger picture of the paragraph. Always go back to the question and make sure you're choosing an answer that actually answers the question and is not just a true statement.

Part IV- Natural Sciences Test Review

These questions will test your knowledge of basic principles and concepts in biology, chemistry, and physics.

While a general knowledge of these subjects is important, a complete mastery of them is NOT necessary to succeed on the Science Test. Don't be intimidated by the questions presented. They do not require highly advanced knowledge, but only the ability to recognize common problem types and apply basic principles and concepts to solving them.

That is our goal, to show you the simple methods to solving these problems, so that while you will not gain a mastery of these subjects from this guide, you will learn the methods necessary to succeed on the exam.

This test may scare you. It may have been years since you've studied some of the basic concepts covered, and for even the most accomplished and studied student, these terms may be unfamiliar. General test-taking skill will help the most. DO NOT run out of time, move quickly, and use the easy pacing methods we outlined in the test-taking tactics section.

The most important thing you can do is to ignore your fears and jump into the test immediately- do not be overwhelmed by any strange-sounding terms. You have to jump into the test like jumping into a pool- all at once is the easiest way. Managing your time on this test can prove to be extremely difficult, as some of the questions may leave you stumped and countless minutes may waste away while you rack your brain for the answer. To be successful though, you must work efficiently and get through the entire test before running out of time.

Scientific Foundations

Scientific Method

One could argue that scientific knowledge is the sum of all scientific inquiries for truths about the natural world carried out throughout the history of human kind. More simply put, it is thanks to scientific inquiry that we know what we do about the world. Scientists use a number of generally accepted techniques collectively known as the scientific method. The scientific method generally involves carrying out the following steps:

- Identifying a problem or posing a question
- Formulating a hypothesis or an educated guess
- Conducting experiments or tests that will provide a basis to solve the problem or answer the question
- Observing the results of the test
- Drawing conclusions

An important part of the scientific method is using acceptable experimentation techniques to ensure results are not skewed. Objectivity is also important if valid results are to be obtained. Another important part of the scientific method is peer review. It is essential that experiments be performed and data be recorded in such a way that experiments can be reproduced to verify results.

A scientific fact is considered an objective and verifiable observation. A scientific theory is a greater body of accepted knowledge, principles, or relationships that might explain a fact. A hypothesis is an educated guess that is not yet proven. It is used to predict the outcome of an experiment in an attempt to solve a problem or answer a question. A law is an explanation of events that always lead to the same outcome. It is a fact that an object falls. The law of gravity explains why an object falls. The theory of relativity, although generally accepted, has been neither proven nor disproved. A model is used to explain something on a smaller scale or in simpler terms to provide an example. It is a representation of an idea that can be used to explain events or applied to new situations to predict outcomes or determine results.

History of Science

When one examines the history of scientific knowledge, it is clear that it is constantly evolving. The body of facts, models, theories, and laws grows and changes over time. In other words, one scientific discovery leads to the next. Some advances in science and technology have important and long-lasting effects on science and society. Some discoveries were so alien to the accepted beliefs of the time that not only were they rejected as wrong, but were also considered outright blasphemy. Today, however, many beliefs once considered incorrect have become an ingrained part of scientific knowledge, and have also been the basis of new advances.

Examples of advances include: Copernicus's heliocentric view of the universe, Newton's laws of motion and planetary orbits, relativity, geologic time scale, plate tectonics, atomic theory, nuclear physics, biological evolution, germ theory, industrial revolution, molecular biology, information and communication, quantum theory, galactic universe, and medical and health technology.

Anton van Leeuwenhoek (d. 1723) used homemade magnifying glasses to become the first person to observe single-celled organisms. He observed bacteria, yeast, plants, and other microscopic organisms. His observations contributed to the field of microbiology.

Carl Linnaeus (d. 1778) created a method to classify plants and animals, which became known as the Linnaean taxonomy. This was an important contribution because it offered a way to organize and therefore study large amounts of data.

Charles Robert Darwin (d. 1882) is best known for contributing to the survival of the fittest through natural selection theory of evolution by observing different species of birds, specifically finches, in various geographic locations. Although the species Darwin looked at were different, he speculated they had a common ancestor. He reasoned that specific traits persisted because they gave the birds a greater chance of surviving and reproducing. He also discovered fossils, noted stratification, dissected marine animals, and interacted with indigenous peoples. He contributed to the fields of biology, marine biology, anthropology, paleontology, geography, and zoology.

Gregor Johann Mendel (d. 1884) is famous for experimenting with pea plants to observe the occurrence of inherited traits. He eventually became known as the father of genetics.

Barbara McClintock (d. 1992) created the first genetic map for maize and was able to demonstrate basic genetic principles, such as how recombination is an exchange of chromosomal information. She also discovered how transposition flips the switch for traits. Her work contributed to the field of genetics, in particular to areas of study concerned with the structure and function of cells and chromosomes.

James Watson and Francis Crick (d. 2004) were co-discoverers of the structure of deoxyribonucleic acid (DNA), which has a double helix shape. DNA contains the code for genetic information. The discovery of the double helix shape was important because it helped to explain how DNA replicates.

Mathematics of Science

Using the metric system is generally accepted as the preferred method for taking measurements. Having a universal standard allows individuals to interpret measurements more easily, regardless of where they are located. The basic units of measurement are: the meter, which measures length; the liter, which measures volume; and the gram, which measures mass. The metric system starts with a base unit and increases or decreases in units of 10. The prefix and the base unit combined are used to indicate an amount. For example, deka is 10 times the base unit. A dekameter is 10 meters; a dekaliter is 10 liters; and a dekagram is 10 grams. The prefix hecto refers to 100 times the base amount; kilo is 1,000 times the base amount. The prefixes that indicate a fraction of the base unit are deci, which is 1/10 of the base unit; centi, which is 1/100 of the base unit; and milli, which is 1/1000 of the base unit.

The mathematical concept of significant figures or significant digits is often used to determine the precision of measurements or the level of confidence one has in a specific measurement. The significant figures of a measurement include all the digits known with certainty plus one estimated or uncertain digit. There are a number of rules for determining which digits are considered "important" or "interesting." They are: all non-zero digits are significant, zeros between digits are significant, and leading and trailing zeros are not significant unless they appear to the right of the non-zero digits in a decimal. For example, in 0.01230 the significant digits are 1230, and this number would be said to be accurate to the hundred-thousandths place. The zero indicates that the amount has actually been measured as 0. Other zeros are considered place holders, and are not important. A decimal point may be placed after zeros to indicate their importance (in 100. for example).

Scientific notation is used because values in science can be very large or very small, which makes them unwieldy. A number in decimal notation is 93,000,000. In scientific notation, it is 9.3 x 107. The first number, 9.3, is the coefficient. It is always greater than or equal to 1 and less than 10. This number is followed by a multiplication sign. The base is always 10 in scientific notation. If the number is greater than ten, the exponent is positive. If the number is between zero and one, the exponent is negative. The first digit of the number is followed by a decimal point and then the rest of the number. In this case, the number is 9.3. To get that number, the decimal point was moved seven places from the end of the number, 93,000,000. The number of places, seven, is the exponent.

Statistics

Data collected during a science lab can be organized and presented in any number of ways. While straight narrative is a suitable method for presenting some lab results, it is not a suitable way to present numbers and quantitative measurements. These types of observations can often be better presented with tables and graphs. Data that is presented in tables and organized in rows and columns may also be used to make graphs quite easily. Other methods of presenting data include illustrations, photographs, video, and even audio formats. In a formal report, tables and figures are labeled and referred to by their labels. For example, a picture of a bubbly solution might be labeled Figure 1, Bubbly Solution. It would be referred to in the text in the following way: "The reaction created bubbles 10 mm in size, as shown in Figure 1, Bubbly Solution." Graphs are also labeled as figures. Tables are labeled in a different way. Examples include: Table 1, Results of Statistical Analysis, or Table 2, Data from Lab 2.

Graphs and charts are effective ways to present scientific data such as observations, statistical analyses, and comparisons between dependent variables and independent variables. On a line chart, the independent variable (the one that is being manipulated for the experiment) is represented on the horizontal axis (the x-axis). Any dependent variables (the ones that may change as the independent variable changes) are represented on the y-axis. The points are charted and a line is drawn to connect the points. An XY or scatter plot is often used to plot many points. A "best fit" line is drawn, which allows outliers to be identified more easily. Charts and their axes should have titles. The x and y interval units should be evenly spaced and labeled. Other types of charts are bar charts and histograms, which can be used to compare differences between the data collected for two variables. A pie chart can graphically show the relation of parts to a whole.

Mean: The mean is the sum of a list of numbers divided by the number of numbers.

Median: If there is an even number of values in the set, the median is calculated by taking the average of the two middle values.

Standard deviation: This measures the variability of a data set and determines the amount of confidence one can have in the conclusions.

Mode: This is the value that appears most frequently in a data set.

Range: This is the difference between the highest and lowest numbers, which can be used to determine how spread out data is.

Regression Analysis: This is a method of analyzing sets of data and sets of variables that involves studying how the typical value of the dependent variable changes when any one of the independent variables is varied and the other independent variables remain fixed.

Earth and Space Science

Geology

Minerals are naturally occurring, inorganic solids with a definite chemical composition and an orderly internal crystal structure. A polymorph is two minerals with the same chemical composition, but a different crystal structure. Rocks are aggregates of one or more minerals, and may also contain mineraloids (minerals lacking a crystalline structure) and organic remains.

The three types of rocks are sedimentary, igneous, and metamorphic. Rocks are classified based on their formation and the minerals they contain. Minerals are classified by their chemical composition. Geology is the study of the planet Earth as it pertains to the composition, structure, and origin of its rocks. Petrology is the study of rocks, including their composition, texture, structure, occurrence, mode of formation, and history. Mineralogy is the study of minerals.

Sedimentary rocks are formed by the process of lithification, which involves compaction, the expulsion of liquids from pores, and the cementation of the pre-existing rock. It is pressure and temperature that are responsible for this process. Sedimentary rocks are often formed in layers in the presence of water, and may contain organic remains, such as fossils. Sedimentary rocks are organized into three groups: detrital, biogenic, and chemical. Texture refers to the size, shape, and grains of sedimentary rock. Texture can be used to determine how a particular sedimentary rock was created. Composition refers to the types of minerals present in the rock. The origin of sedimentary rock refers to the type of water that was involved in its creation. Marine deposits, for example, likely involved ocean environments, while continental deposits likely involved dry land and lakes.

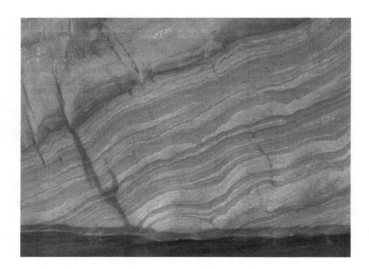

Igneous rock is formed from magma, which is molten material originating from beneath the Earth's surface. Depending upon where magma cools, the resulting igneous rock can be classified as intrusive, plutonic, hypabyssal, extrusive, or volcanic. Magma that solidifies at a depth is intrusive, cools slowly, and has a coarse grain as a result. An example is granite. Magma that solidifies at or near the surface is extrusive, cools quickly, and usually has a fine grain. An example is basalt. Magma that actually flows out of the Earth's surface is called lava. Some extrusive rock cools so quickly that crystals do not have time to form. These rocks have a glassy appearance. An example is obsidian. Hypabyssal rock is igneous rock that is formed at medium depths.

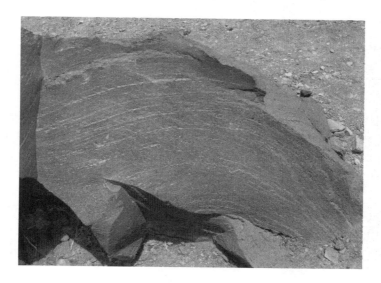

Metamorphic rock is that which has been changed by great heat and pressure. This results in a variety of outcomes, including deformation, compaction, destruction of the characteristics of the original rock, bending, folding, and formation of new minerals because of chemical reactions, and changes in the size and shape of the mineral grain. For example, the igneous rock ferromagnesian can be changed into schist and gneiss. The sedimentary rock carbonaceous can be changed into marble. The texture of metamorphic rocks can be classified as foliated and unfoliated. Foliation, or layering, occurs when rock is compressed along one axis during recrystallization. This can be seen in schist and shale. Unfoliated rock does not include this banding. Rocks that are compressed equally from all sides or lack specific minerals will be unfoliated. An example is marble.

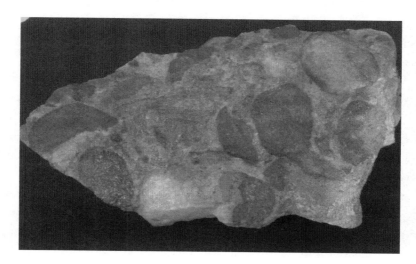

Fossils are preservations of plants, animals, their remains, or their traces that date back to about 10,000 years ago. Fossils and where they are found in rock strata makes up the fossil record. Fossils are formed under a very specific set of conditions. The fossil must not be damaged by predators and scavengers after death, and the fossil must not decompose. Usually, this happens when the organism is quickly covered with sediment. This sediment builds up and molecules in the organism's body are replaced by minerals. Fossils come in an array of sizes, from single-celled organisms to large dinosaurs.

Plate Tectonics

The Earth is ellipsoid, not perfectly spherical. This means the diameter is different through the poles and at the equator. Through the poles, the Earth is about 12,715 km in diameter. The approximate center of the Earth is at a depth of 6,378 km. The Earth is divided into a crust, mantle, and core. The core consists of a solid inner portion. Moving outward, the molten outer core occupies the space from about a depth of 5,150 km to a depth of 2,890 km. The mantle consists of a lower and upper layer. The lower layer includes the D' (D prime) and D" (D double-prime) layers. The solid portion of the upper mantle and crust together form the lithosphere, or rocky sphere. Below this, but still within the mantle, is the asthenosphere, or weak sphere. These layers are distinguishable because the lithosphere is relatively rigid, while the asthenosphere resembles a thick liquid.

The theory of plate tectonics states that the lithosphere, the solid portion of the mantle and Earth's crust, consists of major and minor plates. These plates are on top of and move with the viscous upper mantle, which is heated because of the convection cycle that occurs in the interior of the Earth. There are different estimates as to the exact number of major and minor plates. The number of major plates is believed to be between 9 and 15, and it is thought that there may be as many as 40 minor plates. The United States is atop the North American plate. The Pacific Ocean is atop the Pacific plate. The point at which these two plates slide horizontally along the San Andreas fault is an example of a transform plate boundary. The other two types of boundaries are divergent (plates that are spreading apart and forming new crust) and convergent (the process of subduction causes one plate to go under another). The movement of plates is what causes other features of the Earth's crust, such as mountains, volcanoes, and earthquakes.

Volcanoes can occur along any type of tectonic plate boundary. At a divergent boundary, as plates move apart, magma rises to the surface, cools, and forms a ridge. An example of this is the mid-Atlantic ridge. Convergent boundaries, where one plate slides under another, are often areas with a lot of volcanic activity. The subduction process creates magma. When it rises to the surface, volcanoes can be created. Volcanoes can also be created in the middle of a plate over hot spots. Hot spots are locations where narrow plumes of magma rise through the mantle in a fixed place over a long period of time. The Hawaiian Islands and Midway are examples. The plate shifts and the island moves. Magma continues to rise through the mantle, however, which produces another island. Volcanoes can be active, dormant, or extinct. Active volcanoes are those that are erupting or about to erupt. Dormant volcanoes are those that might erupt in the future and still have internal volcanic activity. Extinct volcanoes are those that will not erupt.

Geography

For the purposes of tracking time and location, the Earth is divided into sections with imaginary lines. Lines that run vertically around the globe through the poles are lines of longitude, sometimes called meridians. The Prime Meridian is the longitudinal reference point of 0. Longitude is measured in 15-degree increments toward the east or west. Degrees are further divided into 60 minutes, and each minute is divided into 60 seconds. Lines of latitude run horizontally around the Earth parallel to the equator, which is the 0 reference point and the widest point of the Earth. Latitude is the distance north or south from the equator, and is also measured in degrees, minutes, and seconds.

Tropic of Cancer: This is located at 23.5 degrees north. The Sun is directly overhead at noon on June 21st in the Tropic of Cancer, which marks the beginning of summer in the Northern Hemisphere.

Tropic of Capricorn: This is located at 23.5 degrees south. The Sun is directly overhead at noon on December 21st in the Tropic of Capricorn, which marks the beginning of winter in the Northern Hemisphere.

Arctic Circle: This is located at 66.5 degrees north, and marks the start of when the Sun is not visible above the horizon. This occurs on December 21st, the same day the Sun is directly over the Tropic of Capricorn.

Antarctic Circle: This is located at 66.5 degrees south, and marks the start of when the Sun is not visible above the horizon. This occurs on June 21st, which marks the beginning of winter in the Southern Hemisphere and is when the Sun is directly over the Tropic of Cancer.

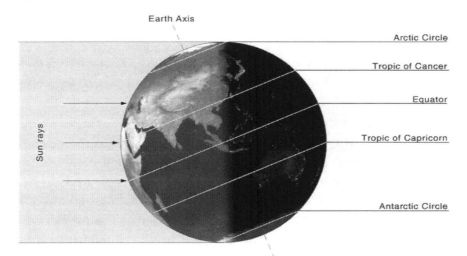

Latitude is a measurement of the distance from the equator. The distance from the equator indicates how much solar radiation a particular area receives. The equator receives more sunlight, while polar areas receive less. The Earth tilts slightly on its rotational axis. This tilt determines the seasons and affects weather. There are eight biomes or ecosystems with particular climates that are associated with latitude. Those in the high latitudes, which get the least sunlight, are tundra and taiga. Those in the mid latitudes are grassland, temperate forest, and chaparral. Those in latitudes closest to the equator are the warmest. The biomes are desert and tropical rain forest. The eighth biome is the ocean, which is unique because it consists of water and spans the entire globe. Insolation refers to incoming solar radiation. Diurnal variations refer to the daily changes in insolation. The greatest insolation occurs at noon.

The tilt of the Earth on its axis is 23.5°. This tilt causes the seasons and affects the temperature because it affects the amount of Sun the area receives. When the Northern or Southern Hemispheres are tilted toward the Sun, the hemisphere tilted toward the sun experiences summer and the other hemisphere experiences winter.

This reverses as the Earth revolves around the Sun. Fall and spring occur between the two extremes. The equator gets the same amount of sunlight every day of the year, about 12 hours, and doesn't experience seasons. Both poles have days during the winter when they are tilted away from the Sun and receive no daylight. The opposite effect occurs during the summer. There are 24 hours of daylight and no night. The summer solstice, the day with the most amount of sunlight, occurs on June 21st in the Northern Hemisphere and on December 21st in the Southern Hemisphere. The winter solstice, the day with the least amount of sunlight, occurs on December 21st in the Northern Hemisphere and on June 21st in the Southern Hemisphere.

Weather, Atmosphere, Water Cycle

Meteorology is the study of the atmosphere, particularly as it pertains to forecasting the weather and understanding its processes. Weather is the condition of the atmosphere at any given moment. Most weather occurs in the troposphere. Weather includes changing events such as clouds, storms, and temperature, as well as more extreme events such as tornadoes, hurricanes, and blizzards. Climate refers to the average weather for a particular area over time, typically at least 30 years. Latitude is an indicator of climate. Changes in climate occur over long time periods.

The hydrologic, or water, cycle refers to water movement on, above, and in the Earth. Water can be in any one of its three states during different phases of the cycle. The three states of water are liquid water, frozen ice, and water vapor. Processes involved in the hydrologic cycle include precipitation, canopy interception, snow melt, runoff, infiltration, subsurface flow, evaporation, sublimation, advection, condensation, and transpiration. Precipitation is when condensed water vapor falls to Earth. Examples include rain, fog drip, and various forms of snow, hail, and sleet. Canopy interception is when precipitation lands on plant foliage instead of falling to the ground and evaporating. Snow melt is runoff produced by melting snow. Infiltration occurs when water flows from the surface into the ground. Subsurface flow refers to water that flows underground. Evaporation is when water in a liquid state changes to a gas. Sublimation is when water in a solid state (such as snow or ice) changes to water vapor without going through a liquid phase. Advection is the movement of water through the atmosphere. Condensation is when water vapor changes to liquid water. Transpiration is when water vapor is released from plants into the air.

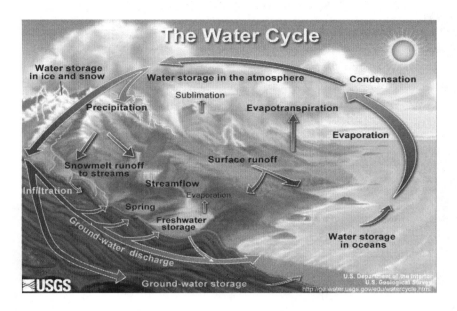

The ocean is the salty body of water that encompasses the Earth. It has a mass of 1.4×10^{24} grams. Geographically, the ocean is divided into three large oceans: the Pacific Ocean, the Atlantic Ocean, and the Indian Ocean. There are also other divisions, such as gulfs, bays, and various types of seas, including Mediterranean and marginal seas. Ocean distances can be measured by latitude, longitude, degrees, meters, miles, and nautical miles. The ocean accounts for 70.8% of the surface of the Earth, amounting to 361,254,000 km². The ocean's depth is greatest at Challenger Deep in the Mariana Trench. The ocean floor here is 10,924 meters below sea level. The depths of the ocean are mapped by echo sounders and satellite altimeter systems. Echo sounders emit a sound pulse from the surface and record the time it takes to return. Satellite altimeters provide better maps of the ocean floor.

The atmosphere consists of 78% nitrogen, 21% oxygen, and 1% argon. It also includes traces of water vapor, carbon dioxide and other gases, dust particles, and chemicals from Earth. The atmosphere becomes thinner the farther it is from the Earth's surface. It becomes difficult to breathe at about 3 km above sea level. The atmosphere gradually fades into space. The lowest layer of the atmosphere is called the troposphere. Its thickness varies at the poles and the equator, varying from about 7 to 17 km. This is where most weather occurs. The stratosphere is next, and continues to an elevation of about 51 km. The mesosphere extends from the stratosphere to an elevation of about 81 km. It is the coldest layer and is where meteors tend to ablate. The next layer is the thermosphere. It is where the International Space Station orbits. The exosphere is the outermost layer, extends to 10,000 km, and mainly consists of hydrogen and helium.

Earth's atmosphere has five main layers. From lowest to highest, these are the troposphere, the stratosphere, the mesosphere, the thermosphere, and the exosphere. Between each pair of layers is a transition layer called a pause. The troposphere includes the tropopause, which is the transitional layer of the stratosphere. Energy from Earth's surface is transferred to the troposphere. Temperature decreases with altitude in this layer. In the stratosphere, the temperature is inverted, meaning that it increases with altitude. The stratosphere includes the ozone layer, which helps block ultraviolet light from the Sun. The stratopause is the transitional layer to the mesosphere. The temperature of the mesosphere decreases with height. It is considered the coldest place on Earth, and has an average temperature of -85 degrees Celsius. Temperature increases with altitude in the thermosphere, which includes the thermopause. Just past the thermosphere is the exobase, the base layer of the exosphere. Beyond the five main layers are the ionosphere, homosphere, heterosphere, and magnetosphere.

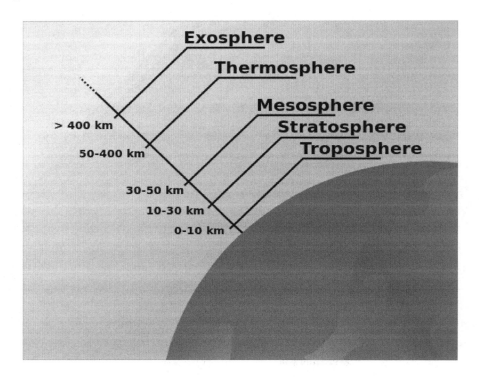

Most clouds can be classified according to the altitude of their base above Earth's surface. High clouds occur at altitudes between 5,000 and 13,000 meters. Middle clouds occur at altitudes between 2,000 and 7,000 meters. Low clouds occur from the Earth's surface to altitudes of 2,000 meters. Types of high clouds include cirrus (Ci), thin wispy mare's tails that consist of ice; cirrocumulus (Cc), small, pillow-like puffs that often appear in rows; and cirrostratus (Cs), thin, sheetlike clouds that often cover the entire sky. Types of middle clouds include altocumulus (Ac), gray-white clouds that consist of liquid water; and altostratus (As), grayish or blue-gray clouds that span the sky. Types of low clouds include stratus (St), gray and fog-like clouds consisting of water droplets that take up the whole sky; stratocumulus (Sc), low-lying, lumpy gray clouds; and nimbostratus (Ns), dark gray clouds with uneven bases that indicate rain or snow. Two types of clouds, cumulus (Cu) and cumulonimbus (Cb), are capable of great vertical growth. They can start at a wide range of altitudes, from the Earth's surface to altitudes of 13,000 meters.

Astronomy

Astronomy is the scientific study of celestial objects and their positions, movements, and structures. Celestial does not refer to the Earth in particular, but does include its motions as it moves through space. Other objects include the Sun, the Moon, planets, satellites, asteroids, meteors, comets, stars, galaxies, the universe, and other space phenomena. The term astronomy has its roots in the Greek words "astro" and "nomos," which means "laws of the stars."

What can be seen of the universe is believed to be at least 93 billion light years across. To put this into perspective, the Milky Way galaxy is about 100,000 light years across. Our view of matter in the universe is that it forms into clumps. Matter is organized into stars, galaxies, clusters of galaxies, superclusters, and the Great Wall of galaxies. Galaxies consist of stars, some with planetary systems. Some estimates state that the universe is about 13 billion years old. It is not considered dense, and is believed to consist of 73 percent dark energy, 23 percent cold dark matter, and 4 percent regular matter. Cosmology is the study of the universe. Interstellar medium (ISM) is the gas and dust in the interstellar space between a galaxy's stars.

The solar system is a planetary system of objects that exist in an ecliptic plane. Objects orbit around and are bound by gravity to a star called the Sun. Objects that orbit around the Sun include: planets, dwarf planets, moons, asteroids, meteoroids, cosmic dust, and comets. The definition of planets has changed. At one time, there were nine planets in the solar system. There are now eight. Planetary objects in the solar system include four inner, terrestrial planets: Mercury, Venus, Earth, and Mars. They are relatively small, dense, rocky, lack rings, and have few or no moons. The four outer, or Jovian, planets are Jupiter, Saturn, Uranus, and Neptune, which are large and have low densities, rings, and moons. They are also known as gas giants. Between the inner and outer planets is the asteroid belt. Beyond Neptune is the Kuiper belt. Within these belts are five dwarf planets: Ceres, Pluto, Haumea, Makemake, and Eris.

The Sun is at the center of the solar system. It is composed of 70% hydrogen (H) and 28% helium (He). The remaining 2% is made up of metals. The Sun is one of 100 billion stars in the Milky Way galaxy. Its diameter is 1,390,000 km, its mass is 1.989×10^{30} kg, its surface temperature is 5,800 K, and its core temperature is 15,600,000 K. The Sun represents more than 99.8% of the total mass of the solar system. At the core, the temperature is 15.6 million K, the pressure is 250 billion atmospheres, and the density is more than 150 times that of water. The surface is called the photosphere. The chromosphere lies above this, and the corona, which extends millions of kilometers into space, is next. Sunspots are relatively cool regions on the surface with a temperature of 3,800 K. Temperatures in the corona are over 1,000,000 K. Its magnetosphere, or heliosphere, extends far beyond Pluto.

Mercury: Mercury is the closest to the Sun and is also the smallest planet. It orbits the Sun every 88 days, has no satellites or atmosphere, has a Moon-like surface with craters, appears bright, and is dense and rocky with a large iron core.

Venus: Venus is the second planet from the Sun. It orbits the Sun every 225 days, is very bright, and is similar to Earth in size, gravity, and bulk composition. It has a dense atmosphere composed of carbon dioxide and some sulfur. It is covered with reflective clouds made of sulfuric acid and exhibits signs of volcanism. Lightning and thunder have been recorded on Venus's surface.

Earth: Earth is the third planet from the Sun. It orbits the Sun every 365 days. Approximately 71% of its surface is salt-water oceans. The Earth is rocky, has an atmosphere composed mainly of oxygen and nitrogen, has one moon, and supports millions of species. It contains the only known life in the solar system.

Mars: Mars it the fourth planet from the Sun. It appears reddish due to iron oxide on the surface, has a thin atmosphere, has a rotational period similar to Earth's, and has seasonal cycles. Surface features of Mars include volcanoes, valleys, deserts, and polar ice caps. Mars has impact craters and the tallest mountain, largest canyon, and perhaps the largest impact crater yet discovered.

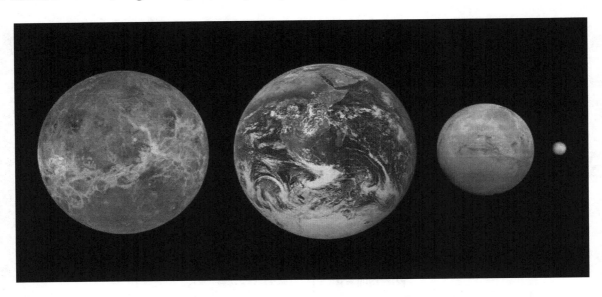

Jupiter: Jupiter is the fifth planet from the Sun and the largest planet in the solar system. It consists mainly of hydrogen, and 25% of its mass is made up of helium. It has a fast rotation and has clouds in the tropopause composed of ammonia crystals that are arranged into bands sub-divided into lighter-hued zones and darker belts causing storms and turbulence. Jupiter has wind speeds of 100 m/s, a planetary ring, 63 moons, and a Great Red Spot, which is an anticyclonic storm.

Saturn: Saturn is the sixth planet from the Sun and the second largest planet in the solar system. It is composed of hydrogen, some helium, and trace elements. Saturn has a small core of rock and ice, a thick layer of metallic hydrogen, a gaseous outer layer, wind speeds of up to 1,800 km/h, a system of rings, and 61 moons.

Uranus: Uranus is the seventh planet from the Sun. Its atmosphere is composed mainly of hydrogen and helium, and also contains water, ammonia, methane, and traces of hydrocarbons. With a minimum temperature of 49 K, Uranus has the coldest atmosphere. Uranus has a ring system, a magnetosphere, and 13 moons.

Neptune: Neptune is the eighth planet from the Sun and is the planet with the third largest mass. It has 12 moons, an atmosphere similar to Uranus, a Great Dark Spot, and the strongest sustained winds of any planet (wind speeds can be as high as 2,100 km/h). Neptune is cold (about 55 K) and has a fragmented ring system.

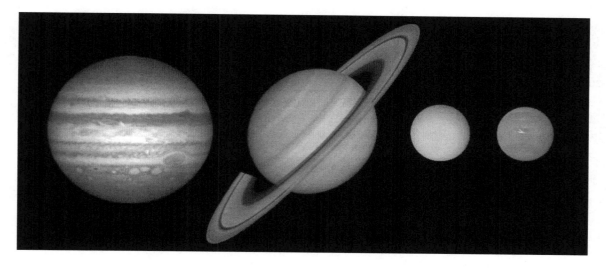

The Earth is about 12,765 km (7,934 miles) in diameter. The Moon is about 3,476 km (2,160 mi) in diameter. The distance between the Earth and the Moon is about 384,401 km (238,910 mi). The diameter of the Sun is approximately 1,390,000 km (866,000 mi). The distance from the Earth to the Sun is 149,598,000 km, also known as 1 Astronomical Unit (AU).

The star that is nearest to the solar system is Proxima Centauri. It is about 270,000 AU away. Some distant galaxies are so far away that their light takes several billion years to reach the Earth. In other words, people on Earth see them as they looked billions of years ago.

It takes about one month for the Moon to go through all its phases. Waxing refers to the two weeks during which the Moon goes from a new moon to a full moon. About two weeks is spent waning, going from a full moon to a new moon. The lit part of the Moon always faces the Sun.

The phases of waxing are: new moon, during which the Moon is not illuminated and rises and sets with the Sun; crescent moon, during which a tiny sliver is lit; first quarter, during which half the Moon is lit and the phase of the Moon is due south on the meridian; gibbous, during which more than half of the Moon is lit and has a shape similar to a football; right side, during which the Moon is lit; and full moon, during which the Moon is fully illuminated, rises at sunset, and sets at sunrise.

After a full moon, the Moon is waning. The phases of waning are: gibbous, during which the left side is lit and the Moon rises after sunset and sets after sunrise; third quarter, during which the Moon is half lit and rises at midnight and sets at noon; crescent, during which a tiny sliver is lit; and new moon, during which the Moon is not illuminated and rises and sets with the Sun.

Biology

Cells

The main difference between eukaryotic and prokaryotic cells is that eukaryotic cells have a nucleus and prokaryotic cells do not. Eukaryotic cells are considered more complex, while prokaryotic cells are smaller and simpler. Eukaryotic cells have membrane-bound organelles that perform various functions and contribute to the complexity of these types of cells. Prokaryotic cells do not contain membrane-bound organelles. In prokaryotic cells, the genetic material (DNA) is not contained within a membrane-bound nucleus. Instead, it aggregates in the cytoplasm in a nucleoid. In eukaryotic cells, DNA is mostly contained in chromosomes in the nucleus, although there is some DNA in mitochondria and chloroplasts. Prokaryotic cells usually divide by binary fission and are haploid. Eukaryotic cells divide by mitosis and are diploid. Prokaryotic structures include plasmids, ribosomes, cytoplasm, a cytoskeleton, granules of nutritional substances, a plasma membrane, flagella, and a few others. They are single-celled organisms. Bacteria are prokaryotic cells.

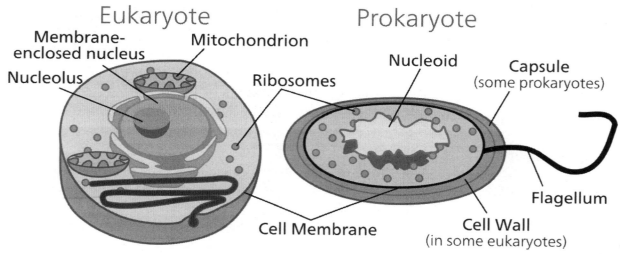

The functions of plant and animal cells vary greatly, and the functions of different cells within a single organism can also be vastly different. Animal and plant cells are similar in structure in that they are eukaryotic, which means they contain a nucleus. The nucleus is a round structure that controls the activities of the cell and contains chromosomes. Both types of cells have cell membranes, cytoplasm, vacuoles, and other structures. The main difference between the two is that plant cells have a cell wall made of cellulose that can handle high levels of pressure within the cell, which can occur when liquid enters a plant cell. Plant cells have chloroplasts that are used during the process of photosynthesis, which is the conversion of sunlight into food. Plant cells usually have one large vacuole, whereas animal cells can have many smaller ones. Plant cells have a regular shape, while the shapes of animal cell can vary.

Plant cells can be much larger than animal cells, ranging from 10 to 100 micrometers. Animal cells are 10 to 30 micrometers in size. Plant cells can have much larger vacuoles that occupy a large portion of the cell. They also have cell walls, which are thick barriers consisting of protein and sugars. Animal cells lack cell walls. Chloroplasts in plants that perform photosynthesis absorb sunlight and convert it into energy. Mitochondria produce energy from food in animal cells. Plant and animal cells are both eukaryotic, meaning they contain a nucleus. Both plant and animal cells duplicate genetic material, separate it, and then divide in half to reproduce. Plant cells build a cell plate between the two new cells, while animal cells make a cleavage furrow and pinch in half. Microtubules are components of the cytoskeleton in both plant and animal cells. Microtubule organizing centers (MTOCs) make microtubules in plant cells, while centrioles make microtubules in animal cells.

Photosynthesis is the conversion of sunlight into energy in plant cells, and also occurs in some types of bacteria and protists. Carbon dioxide and water are converted into glucose during photosynthesis, and light is required during this process. Cyanobacteria are thought to be the descendants of the first organisms to use photosynthesis about 3.5 billion years ago. Photosynthesis is a form of cellular respiration. It occurs in chloroplasts that use thylakoids, which are structures in the membrane that contain light reaction chemicals. Chlorophyll is a pigment that absorbs light. During the process, water is used and oxygen is released. The equation for the chemical reaction that occurs during photosynthesis is $6H_2O + 6CO_2 \rightarrow C_6H_{12}O_6 + 6O_2$. During photosynthesis, six molecules of water and six molecules of carbon dioxide react to form one molecule of sugar and six molecules of oxygen.

The term cell cycle refers to the process by which a cell reproduces, which involves cell growth, the duplication of genetic material, and cell division. Complex organisms with many cells use the cell cycle to replace cells as they lose their functionality and wear out. The entire cell cycle in animal cells can take 24 hours. The time required varies among different cell types. Human skin cells, for example, are constantly reproducing. Some other cells only divide infrequently. Once neurons are mature, they do not grow or divide. The two ways that cells can reproduce are through meiosis and mitosis. When cells replicate through mitosis, the "daughter cell" is an exact replica of the parent cell. When cells divide through meiosis, the daughter cells have different genetic coding than the parent cell. Meiosis only happens in specialized reproductive cells called gametes.

Mitosis is the process of cell reproduction in which a eukaryotic cell splits into two separate, but completely identical, cells. This process is divided into a number of different phases.

Interphase: The cell prepares for division by replicating its genetic and cytoplasmic material. Interphase can be further divided into G1, S, and G2.

Prophase: The chromatin thickens into chromosomes and the nuclear membrane begins to disintegrate. Pairs of centrioles move to opposite sides of the cell and spindle fibers begin to form. The mitotic spindle, formed from cytoskeleton parts, moves chromosomes around within the cell.

Metaphase: The spindle moves to the center of the cell and chromosome pairs align along the center of the spindle structure.

Anaphase: The pairs of chromosomes, called sisters, begin to pull apart, and may bend. When they are separated, they are called daughter chromosomes. Grooves appear in the cell membrane.

Telophase: The spindle disintegrates, the nuclear membranes reform, and the chromosomes revert to chromatin. In animal cells, the membrane is pinched. In plant cells, a new cell wall begins to form.

Cytokinesis: This is the physical splitting of the cell (including the cytoplasm) into two cells. Some believe this occurs following telophase. Others say it occurs from anaphase, as the cell begins to furrow, through telophase, when the cell actually splits into two.

Meiosis is another process by which eukaryotic cells reproduce. However, meiosis is used by more complex life forms such as plants and animals and results in four unique cells rather than two identical cells as in mitosis. Meiosis has the same phases as mitosis, but they happen twice. In addition, different events occur during some phases of meiosis than mitosis. The events that occur during the first phase of meiosis are interphase (I), prophase (I), metaphase (I), anaphase (I), telophase (I), and cytokinesis (I). During this first phase of meiosis, chromosomes cross over, genetic material is exchanged, and tetrads of four chromatids are formed. The nuclear membrane dissolves. Homologous pairs of chromatids are separated and travel to different poles. At this point, there has been one cell division resulting in two cells. Each cell goes through a second cell division, which consists of prophase (II), metaphase (II), anaphase (II), telophase (II), and cytokinesis (II). The result is four daughter cells with different sets of chromosomes. The daughter cells are haploid, which means they contain half the genetic material of the parent cell. The second phase of meiosis is similar to the process of mitosis. Meiosis encourages genetic diversity.

Genetics

Chromosomes consist of genes, which are single units of genetic information. Genes are made up of deoxyribonucleic acid (DNA). DNA is a nucleic acid located in the cell nucleus. There is also DNA in the mitochondria. DNA replicates to pass on genetic information. The DNA in almost all cells is the same. It is also involved in the biosynthesis of proteins. The model or structure of DNA is described as a double helix. A helix is a curve, and a double helix is two congruent curves connected by horizontal members. The model can be likened to a spiral staircase. It is right-handed. The British scientist Rosalind Elsie Franklin is credited with taking the x-ray diffraction image in 1952 that was used by Francis Crick and James Watson to formulate the double-helix model of DNA and speculate about its important role in carrying and transferring genetic information.

DNA has a double helix shape, resembles a twisted ladder, and is compact. It consists of nucleotides. Nucleotides consist of a five-carbon sugar (pentose), a phosphate group, and a nitrogenous base. Two bases pair up to form the rungs of the ladder. The "side rails" or backbone consists of the covalently bonded sugar and phosphate. The bases are attached to each other with hydrogen bonds, which are easily dismantled so replication can occur. Each base is attached to a phosphate and to a sugar. There are four types of nitrogenous bases: adenine (A), guanine (G), cytosine (C), and thymine (T). There are about 3 billion bases in human DNA. The bases are mostly the same in everybody, but their order is different. It is the order of these bases that creates diversity in people. Adenine (A) pairs with thymine (T), and cytosine (C) pairs with guanine (G).

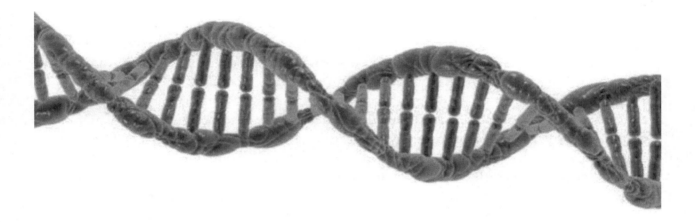

A gene is a portion of DNA that identifies how traits are expressed and passed on in an organism. A gene is part of the genetic code. Collectively, all genes form the genotype of an individual. The genotype includes genes that may not be expressed, such as recessive genes. The phenotype is the physical, visual manifestation of genes. It is determined by the basic genetic information and how genes have been affected by their environment. An allele is a variation of a gene. Also known as a trait, it determines the manifestation of a gene. This manifestation results in a specific physical appearance of some facet of an organism, such as eye color or height. For example the genetic information for eye color is a gene. The gene variations responsible for blue, green, brown, or black eyes are called alleles. Locus (pl. loci) refers to the location of a gene or alleles.

Mendel's laws are the law of segregation (the first law) and the law of independent assortment (the second law). The law of segregation states that there are two alleles and that half of the total number of alleles are contributed by each parent organism. The law of independent assortment states that traits are passed on randomly and are not influenced by other traits. The exception to this is linked traits. A Punnett square can illustrate how alleles combine from the contributing genes to form various phenotypes. One set of a parent's genes are put in columns, while the genes from the other parent are placed in rows. The allele combinations are shown in each cell. When two different alleles are present in a pair, the dominant one is expressed. A Punnett square can be used to predict the outcome of crosses.

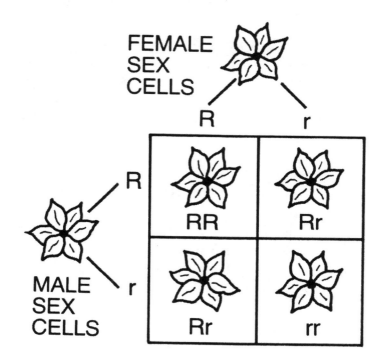

Gene traits are represented in pairs with an upper case letter for the dominant trait (A) and a lower case letter for the recessive trait (a). Genes occur in pairs (AA, Aa, or aa). There is one gene on each chromosome half supplied by each parent organism. Since half the genetic material is from each parent, the offspring's traits are represented as a combination of these. A dominant trait only requires one gene of a gene pair for it to be expressed in a phenotype, whereas a recessive requires both genes in order to be manifested. For example, if the mother's genotype is Dd and the father's is dd, the possible combinations are Dd and dd. The dominant trait will be manifested if the genotype is DD or Dd. The recessive trait will be manifested if the genotype is dd. Both DD and dd are homozygous pairs. Dd is heterozygous.

Evolution

Scientific evidence supporting the theory of evolution can be found in biogeography, comparative anatomy and embryology, the fossil record, and molecular evidence. Biogeography studies the geographical distribution of animals and plants. Evidence of evolution related to the area of biogeography includes species that are well suited for extreme environments. The fossil record shows that species lived only for a short time period before becoming extinct. The fossil record can also show the succession of plants and animals. Living fossils are existing species that have not changed much morphologically and are very similar to ancient examples in the fossil record. Examples include the horseshoe crab and gingko. Comparative embryology studies how species are similar in the embryonic stage, but become increasingly specialized and diverse as they age. Vestigial organs are those that still exist, but become nonfunctional. Examples include the hind limbs of whales and the wings of birds that can no longer fly, such as ostriches.

The rate of evolution is affected by the variability of a population. Variability increases the likelihood of evolution. Variability in a population can be increased by mutations, immigration, sexual reproduction (as opposed to asexual reproduction), and size. Natural selection, emigration, and smaller populations can lead to decreased variability. Sexual selection affects evolution. If fewer genes are available, it will limit the number of genes passed on to subsequent generations. Some animal mating behaviors are not as successful as others. A male that does not attract a female because of a weak mating call or dull feathers, for example, will not pass on its genes. Mechanical isolation, which refers to sex organs that do not fit together very well, can also decrease successful mating.

Natural selection: This theory developed by Darwin states that traits that help give a species a survival advantage are passed on to subsequent generations. Members of a species that do not have the advantageous trait die before they reproduce. Darwin's four principles are: from generation to generation, there are various individuals within a species; genes determine variations; more individuals are born than survive to maturation; and specific genes enable an organism to better survive.

Gradualism: This can be contrasted with punctuationism. It is an idea that evolution proceeds at a steady pace and does not include sudden developments of new species or features from one generation to the next.

Punctuated Equilibrium: This can be contrasted with gradualism. It is the idea in evolutionary biology that states that evolution involves long time periods of no change (stasis) accompanied by relatively brief periods (hundreds of thousands of years) of rapid change.

Three types of evolution are divergent, convergent, and parallel. Divergent evolution refers to two species that become different over time. This can be caused by one of the species adapting to a different environment. Convergent evolution refers to two species that start out fairly different, but evolve to share many similar traits. Parallel evolution refers to species that are not similar and do not become more or less similar over time. Mechanisms of evolution include descent (the passing on of genetic information), mutation, migration, natural selection, and genetic variation and drift. The biological definition of species refers to a group of individuals that can mate and reproduce. Speciation refers to the evolution of a new biological species. The biological species concept (BSC) basically states that a species is a community of individuals that can reproduce and have a niche in nature.

One theory of how life originated on Earth is that life developed from nonliving materials. The first stage of this transformation happened when abiotic (nonliving) synthesis took place, which is the formation of monomers like amino acids and nucleotides. Next, monomers joined together to create polymers such as proteins and nucleic acids. These polymers are then believed to have formed into protobionts. The last stage was the development of the process of heredity. Supporters of this theory believe that RNA was the first genetic material. Another theory postulates that hereditary systems came about before the origination of nucleic acids. Another theory is that life, or the precursors for it, were transported to Earth from a meteorite or other object from space. There is no real evidence to support this theory.

A number of scientists have made significant contributions to the theory of evolution:

Cuvier (1744-1829): Cuvier was a French naturalist who used the fossil record (paleontology) to compare the anatomies of extinct species and existing species to make conclusions about extinction. He believed in the catastrophism theory more strongly than the theory of evolution.

Lamarck (1769-1832): Lamarck was a French naturalist who believed in the idea of evolution and thought it was a natural occurrence influenced by the environment. He studied medicine and botany. Lamarck put forth a theory of evolution by inheritance of acquired characteristics. He theorized that organisms became more complex by moving up a ladder of progress.

Lyell (1797-1875): Lyell was a British geologist who believed in geographical uniformitarianism, which can be contrasted with catastrophism.

Charles Robert Darwin (1809-1882): Darwin was an English naturalist known for his belief that evolution occurred by natural selection. He believed that species descend from common ancestors.

Alfred Russell Wallace (1823-1913): He was a British naturalist who independently developed a theory of evolution by natural selection. He believed in the transmutation of species (that one species develops into another).

Organism Classification

The groupings in the five kingdom classification system are kingdom, phylum/division, class, order, family, genus, and species. A memory aid for this is: King Phillip Came Over For Good Soup. The five kingdoms are Monera, Protista, Fungi, Plantae, and Animalia. The kingdom is the top level classification in this system. Below that are the following groupings: phylum, class, order, family, genus, and species. The Monera kingdom includes about 10,000 known species of prokaryotes, such as bacteria and cyanobacteria. Members of this kingdom can be unicellular organisms or colonies. The next four kingdoms consist of eukaryotes. The Protista kingdom includes about 250,000 species of unicellular protozoans and unicellular and multicellular algae. The Fungi kingdom includes about 100,000 species. A recently introduced system of classification includes a three domain grouping above kingdom. The domain groupings are Archaea, Bacteria (which both consist of prokaryotes), and Eukarya, which include eukaryotes. According to the five kingdom classification system, humans are: kingdom Animalia, phylum Chordata, subphylum Vertebrata, class Mammalia, order Primate, family Hominidae, genus Homo, and species Sapiens.

An organism is a living thing. A unicellular organism is an organism that has only one cell. Examples of unicellular organisms are bacteria and paramecium. A multicellular organism is one that consists of many cells. Humans are a good example. By some estimates, the human body is made up of billions of cells. Others think the human body has more than 75 trillion cells. The term microbe refers to small organisms that are only visible through a microscope. Examples include viruses, bacteria, fungi, and protozoa. Microbes are also referred to as microorganisms, and it is these that are studied by microbiologists. Bacteria can be rod shaped, round (cocci), or spiral (spirilla). These shapes are used to differentiate among types of bacteria. Bacteria can be identified by staining them. This particular type of stain is called a gram stain. If bacteria are gram-positive, they absorb the stain and become purple. If bacteria are gram-negative, they do not absorb the stain and become a pinkish color.

Organisms in the Protista kingdom are classified according to their methods of locomotion, their methods of reproduction, and how they get their nutrients. Protists can move by the use of a flagellum, cilia, or pseudopod. Flagellates have flagellum, which are long tails or whip-like structures that are rotated to help the protist move. Ciliates use cilia, which are smaller hair-like structures on the exterior of a cell that wiggle to help move the surrounding matter. Amoeboids use pseudopodia to move. Bacteria reproduce either sexually or asexually. Binary fission is a form of asexual reproduction whereby bacteria divide in half to produce two new organisms that are clones of the parent. In sexual reproduction, genetic material is exchanged. When kingdom members are categorized according to how they obtain nutrients, the three types of protists are photosynthetic, consumers, and saprophytes. Photosynthetic protists convert sunlight into energy. Organisms that use photosynthesis are considered producers. Consumers, also known as heterotrophs, eat or consume other organisms. Saprophytes consume dead or decaying substances.

Mycology is the study of fungi. The Fungi kingdom includes about 100,000 species. They are further delineated as mushrooms, yeasts, molds, rusts, mildews, stinkhorns, puffballs, and truffles. Fungi are characterized by cell walls that have chitin, a long chain polymer carbohydrate. Fungi are different from species in the Plant kingdom, which have cell walls consisting of cellulose. Fungi are thought to have evolved from a single ancestor. Although they are often thought of as a type of plant, they are more similar to animals than plants. Fungi are typically small and numerous, and have a diverse morphology among species. They can have bright red cups and be orange jellylike masses, and their shapes can resemble golf balls, bird nests with eggs, starfish, parasols, and male genitalia. Some members of the stinkhorn family emit odors similar to dog scat to attract flies that help transport spores that are involved in reproduction. Fungi of this family are also consumed by humans.

Chlorophyta are green algae. Bryophyta are nonvascular mosses and liverworts. They have root-like parts called rhizoids. Since they do not have the vascular structures to transport water, they live in moist environments. Lycophyta are club mosses. They are vascular plants. They use spores and need water to reproduce. Equisetopsida (sphenophyta) are horsetails. Like lycophyta, they need water to reproduce with spores. They have rhizoids and needle-like leaves. The pteridophytes (filicopsida) are ferns. They have stems (rhizomes). Spermatopsida are the seed plants. Gymnosperms are a conifer, which means they have cones with seeds that are used in reproduction. Plants with seeds require less water. Cycadophyta are cone-bearing and look like palms. Gnetophyta are plants that live in the desert. Coniferophyta are pine trees, and have both cones and needles. Ginkgophyta are ginkos. Anthophyta is the division with the largest number of plant species, and includes flowering plants with true seeds.

Only plants in the division bryophyta (mosses and liverworts) are nonvascular, which means they do not have xylem to transport water. All of the plants in the remaining divisions are vascular, meaning they have true roots, stems, leaves, and xylem. Pteridophytes are plants that use spores and not seeds to reproduce. They include the following divisions: Psilophyta (whisk fern), Lycophyta (club mosses), Sphenophyta (horsetails), and Pterophyta (ferns). Spermatophytes are plants that use seeds to reproduce. Included in this category are gymnosperms, which are flowerless plants that use naked seeds, and angiosperms, which are flowering plants that contain seeds in or on a fruit. Gymnosperms include the following divisions: cycadophyta (cycads), ginkgophyta (maidenhair tree), gnetophyta (ephedra and welwitschia), and coniferophyta (which includes pinophyta conifers). Angiosperms comprise the division anthophyta (flowering plants).

Plants are autotrophs, which mean they make their own food. In a sense, they are self sufficient. Three major processes used by plants are photosynthesis, transpiration, and respiration. Photosynthesis involves using sunlight to make food for plants. Transpiration evaporates water out of plants. Respiration is the utilization of food that was produced during photosynthesis.

Two major systems in plants are the shoot and the root system. The shoot system includes leaves, buds, and stems. It also includes the flowers and fruits in flowering plants. The shoot system is located above the ground. The root system is the component of the plant that is underground, and includes roots, tubers, and rhizomes. Meristems form plant cells by mitosis. Cells then differentiate into cell types to form the three types of plant tissues, which are dermal, ground, and vascular. Dermal refers to tissues that form the covering or outer layer of a plant. Ground tissues consist of parenchyma, collenchyma, and/or sclerenchyma cells.

There are at least 230,000 species of flowering plants. They represent about 90 percent of all plants. Angiosperms have a sexual reproduction phase that includes flowering. When growing plants, one may think they develop in the following order: seeds, growth, flowers, and fruit. The reproductive cycle has the following order: flowers, fruit, and seeds. In other words, seeds are the products of successful reproduction. The colors and scents of flowers serve to attract pollinators. Flowers and other plants can also be pollinated by wind. When a pollen grain meets the ovule and is successfully fertilized, the ovule develops into a seed. A seed consists of three parts: the embryo, the endosperm, and a seed coat. The embryo is a small plant that has started to develop, but this development is paused. Germination is when the embryo starts to grow again. The endosperm consists of proteins, carbohydrates, or fats. It typically serves as a food source for the embryo. The seed coat provides protection from disease, insects, and water.

The animal kingdom is comprised of more than one million species in about 30 divisions (the plant kingdom uses the term phyla). There about 800,000 species of insects alone, representing half of all animal species. The characteristics that distinguish members of the animal kingdom from members of other kingdoms are that they are multicellular, are heterotrophic, reproduce sexually (there are some exceptions), have cells that do not contain cell walls or photosynthetic pigments, can move at some stage of life, and can rapidly respond to the environment as a result of specialized tissues like nerve and muscle. Heterotrophic refers to the method of getting energy by eating food that has energy releasing substances. Plants, on the other hand, are autotrophs, which mean they make their own energy. During reproduction, animals have a diploid embryo in the blastula stage. This structure is unique to animals. The blastula resembles a fluid-filled ball.

The animal kingdom includes about one million species. Metazoans are multicellular animals. Food is ingested and enters a mesoderm-lined coelom (body cavity). Phylum porifera and coelenterate are exceptions. The taxonomy of animals involves grouping them into phyla according to body symmetry and plan, as well as the presence of or lack of segmentation. The more complex phyla that have a coelom and a digestive system are further classified as protostomes or deuterostomes according to blastula development. In protostomes, the blastula's blastopore (opening) forms a mouth. In deuterostomes, the blastopore forms an anus. Taxonomy schemes vary, but there are about 36 phyla of animals. The corresponding term for plants at this level is division. The most notable phyla include chordata, mollusca, porifera, cnidaria, platyhelminthes, nematoda, annelida, arthropoda, and echinodermata, which account for about 96 percent of all animal species.

These four animal phyla lack a coelom or have a pseudocoelom.

Porifera: These are sponges. They lack a coelom and get food as water flows through them. They are usually found in marine and sometimes in freshwater environments. They are perforated and diploblastic, meaning there are two layers of cells.

Cnidaria: Members of this phylum are hydrozoa, jellyfish, and obelia. They have radial symmetry, sac-like bodies, and a polyp or medusa (jellyfish) body plan. They are diploblastic, possessing both an ectoderm and an endoderm. Food can get in through a cavity, but members of this phylum do not have an anus.

Platyhelminthes: These are also known as flatworms. Classes include turbellaria (planarian) and trematoda (which include lung, liver, and blood fluke parasites). They have organs and bilateral symmetry. They have three layers of tissue: an ectoderm, a mesoderm, and an endoderm.

Nematoda: These are roundworms. Hookworms and many other parasites are members of this phylum. They have a pseudocoelom, which means the coelom is not completely enclosed within the mesoderm. They also have a digestive tract that runs directly from the mouth to the anus. They are nonsegmented.

Members of the protostomic phyla have mouths that are formed from blastopores.

Mollusca: Classes include bivalvia (organisms with two shells, such as clams, mussels, and oysters), gastropoda (snails and slugs), cephalopoda (octopus, squid, and chambered nautilus), scaphopoda, amphineura (chitons), and monoplacophora.

Annelida: This phylum includes the classes oligochaeta (earthworms), polychaeta (clam worms), and hirudinea (leeches). They have true coeloms enclosed within the mesoderm. They are segmented, have repeating units, and have a nerve trunk.

Arthropoda: The phylum is diverse and populous. Members can be found in all types of environments. They have external skeletons, jointed appendages, bilateral symmetry, and nerve cords. They also have open circulatory systems and sense organs. Subphyla include crustacea (lobster, barnacles, pill bugs, and daphnia), hexapoda (all insects, which have three body segments, six legs, and usual wings), myriapoda (centipedes and millipedes), and chelicerata (the horseshoe crab and arachnids). Pill bugs have gills. Bees, ants, and wasps belong to the order hymenoptera. Like several other insect orders, they undergo complete metamorphosis.

Members of the deuterostomic phyla have anuses that are formed from blastopores.

Echinodermata: Members of this phylum have radial symmetry, are marine organisms, and have a water vascular system. Classes include echinoidea (sea urchins and sand dollars), crinoidea (sea lilies), asteroidea (starfish), ophiuroidea (brittle stars), and holothuroidea (sea cucumbers).

Chordata: This phylum includes humans and all other vertebrates, as well as a few invertebrates (urochordata and cephalochordata). Members of this phylum include agnatha (lampreys and hagfish), gnathostomata, chondrichthyes (cartilaginous fish-like sharks, skates, and rays), osteichthyes (bony fishes, including ray-finned fish that humans eat), amphibians (frogs, salamander, and newts), reptiles (lizards, snakes, crocodiles, and dinosaurs), birds, and mammals.

Anatomy

Extrinsic refers to homeostatic systems that are controlled from outside the body. In higher animals, the nervous system and endocrine system help regulate body functions by responding to stimuli. Hormones in animals regulate many processes, including growth, metabolism, reproduction, and fluid balance. The names of hormones tend to end in "-one." Endocrine hormones are proteins or steroids. Steroid hormones (anabolic steroids) help control the manufacture of protein in muscles and bones.

Invertebrates do not have a backbone, whereas vertebrates do. The great majority of animal species (an estimated 98 percent) are invertebrates, including worms, jellyfish, mollusks, slugs, insects, and spiders. They comprise 30 phyla in all. Vertebrates belong to the phylum chordata. The vertebrate body has two cavities. The thoracic cavity holds the heart and lungs and the abdominal cavity holds the digestive organs. Animals with exoskeletons have skeletons on the outside. Examples are crabs and turtles. Animals with endoskeletons have skeletons on the inside. Examples are humans, tigers, birds, and reptiles.

The 11 major organ systems are: skeletal, muscular, nervous, digestive, respiratory, circulatory, skin, excretory, immune, endocrine, and reproductive.

Skeletal: This consists of the bones and joints. The skeletal system provides support for the body through its rigid structure, provides protection for internal organs, and works to make organisms motile. Growth hormone affects the rate of reproduction and the size of body cells, and also helps amino acids move through membranes.

Muscular: This includes the muscles. The muscular system allows the body to move and respond to its environment.

Nervous: This includes the brain, spinal cord, and nerves. The nervous system is a signaling system for intrabody communications among systems, responses to stimuli, and interaction within an environment. Signals are electrochemical. Conscious thoughts and memories and sense interpretation occur in the nervous system. It also controls involuntary muscles and functions, such as breathing and the beating of the heart.

> ➤ **Review Video: <u>Nervous System</u>**
> *Visit **mometrix.com/academy** and enter **Code: 708428***

Digestive: This includes the mouth, pharynx, esophagus, stomach, intestines, rectum, anal canal, teeth, salivary glands, tongue, liver, gallbladder, pancreas, and appendix. The system helps change food into a form that the body can process and use for energy and nutrients. Food is eventually eliminated as solid waste. Digestive processes can be mechanical, such as chewing food and churning it in the stomach, and chemical, such as secreting hydrochloric acid to kill bacteria and converting protein to amino acids. The overall system converts large food particles into molecules so the body can use them. The small intestine transports the molecules to the circulatory system. The large intestine absorbs nutrients and prepares the unused portions of food for elimination.

Carbohydrates are the primary source of energy as they can be easily converted to glucose. Fats (oils or lipids) are usually not very water soluble, and vitamins A, D, E, and K are fat soluble. Fats are needed to help process these vitamins and can also store energy. Fats have the highest calorie value per gram (9,000 calories). Dietary fiber, or roughage, helps the excretory system. In humans, fiber can help regulate blood sugar levels, reduce heart disease, help food pass through the digestive system, and add bulk. Dietary minerals are chemical elements that are involved with biochemical functions in the body. Proteins consist of amino acids. Proteins are broken down in the body into amino acids that are used for protein biosynthesis or fuel. Vitamins are compounds that are not made by the body, but obtained through the diet. Water is necessary to prevent dehydration since water is lost through the excretory system and perspiration.

Respiratory: This includes the nose, pharynx, larynx, trachea, bronchi, and lungs. It is involved in gas exchange, which occurs in the alveoli. Fish have gills instead of lungs.

Circulatory: This includes the heart, blood, and blood vessels, such as veins, arteries, and capillaries. Blood transports oxygen and nutrients to cells and carbon dioxide to the lungs.

Skin (integumentary): This includes skin, hair, nails, sense receptors, sweat glands, and oil glands. The skin is a sense organ, provides an exterior barrier against disease, regulates body temperature through perspiration, manufactures chemicals and hormones, and provides a place for nerves from the nervous system and parts of the circulation system to travel through. Skin has three layers: epidermis, dermis, and subcutaneous. The epidermis is the thin, outermost, waterproof layer. Basal cells are located in the epidermis. The dermis contains the sweat glands, oil glands, and hair follicles. The subcutaneous layer has connective tissue, and also contains adipose (fat) tissue, nerves, arteries, and veins.

Excretory: This includes the kidneys, ureters, bladder, and urethra. The excretory system helps maintain the amount of fluids in the body. Wastes from the blood system and excess water are removed in urine. The system also helps remove solid waste.

Immune: This includes the lymphatic system, lymph nodes, lymph vessels, thymus, and spleen. Lymph fluid is moved throughout the body by lymph vessels that provide protection against disease. This system protects the body from external intrusions, such as microscopic organisms and foreign substances. It can also protect against some cancerous cells.

Endocrine: This includes the pituitary gland, pineal gland, hypothalamus, thyroid gland, parathyroids, thymus, adrenals, pancreas, ovaries, and testes. It controls systems and processes by secreting hormones into the blood system. Exocrine glands are those that secrete fluid into ducts. Endocrine glands secrete hormones directly into the blood stream without the use of ducts. Prostaglandin (tissue hormones) diffuses only a short distance from the tissue that created it, and influences nearby cells only. Adrenal glands are located above each kidney. The cortex secretes some sex hormones, as well as mineralocorticoids and glucocorticoids involved in immune suppression and stress response. The medulla secretes epinephrine and norepinephrine. Both elevate blood sugar, increase blood pressure, and accelerate heart rate. Epinephrine also stimulates heart muscle. The islets of Langerhans are clumped within the pancreas and secrete glucagon and insulin, thereby regulating blood sugar levels. The four parathyroid glands at the rear of the thyroid secrete parathyroid hormone.

Reproductive: In the male, this system includes the testes, vas deferens, urethra, prostate, penis, and scrotum. In the female, this system includes the ovaries, fallopian tubes (oviduct and uterine tubes), cervix, uterus, vagina, vulva, and mammary glands. Sexual reproduction helps provide genetic diversity as gametes from each parent contribute half the DNA to the zygote offspring. The system provides a method of transporting the male gametes to the female. It also allows for the growth and development of the embryo. Hormones involved are testosterone, interstitial cell stimulating hormone (ICSH), luteinizing hormone (LH), follicle stimulating hormone (FSH), and estrogen. Estrogens secreted from the ovaries include estradiol, estrone, and estriol. They encourage growth, among other things. Progesterone helps prepare the endometrium for pregnancy.

Based on whether or not and when an organism uses meiosis or mitosis, the three possible cycles of reproduction are haplontic, diplontic, and haplodiplontic. Fungi, green algae, and protozoa are haplontic. Animals and some brown algae and fungi are diplontic. Plants and some fungi are haplodiplontic. Diplontic organisms, like multicelled animals, have a dominant diploid life cycle. The haploid generation is simply the egg and sperm. Monoecious species are bisexual (hermaphroditic). In this case, the individual has both male and female organs: sperm-bearing testicles and egg-bearing ovaries. Hermaphroditic species can self fertilize. Some worms are hermaphroditic. Cross fertilization is when individuals exchange genetic information. Most animal species are dioecious, meaning individuals are distinctly male or female.

Biological Relationships

As heterotrophs, animals can be further classified as carnivores, herbivores, omnivores, and parasites. Predation refers to a predator that feeds on another organism, which results in its death. Detritivory refers to heterotrophs that consume organic dead matter. Carnivores are animals that are meat eaters. Herbivores are plant eaters, and omnivores eat both meat and plants. A parasite's food source is its host. A parasite lives off of a host, which does not benefit from the interaction. Nutrients can be classified as carbohydrates, fats, fiber, minerals, proteins, vitamins, and water. Each supply a specific substance required for various species to survive, grow, and reproduce. A calorie is a measurement of heat energy. It can be used to represent both how much energy a food can provide and how much energy an organism needs to live.

Biochemical cycles are how chemical elements required by living organisms cycle between living and nonliving organisms. Elements that are frequently required are phosphorus, sulfur, oxygen, carbon, gaseous nitrogen, and water. Elements can go through gas cycles, sedimentary cycles, or both. Elements circulate through the air in a gas cycle and from land to water in a sedimentary one.

A food chain is a linking of organisms in a community that is based on how they use each other as food sources. Each link in the chain consumes the link above it and is consumed by the link below it. The exceptions are the organism at the top of the food chain and the organism at the bottom.

Biomagnification (bioamplification): This refers to an increase in concentration of a substance within a food chain. Examples are pesticides or mercury. Mercury is emitted from coal-fired power plants and gets into the water supply, where it is eaten by a fish. A larger fish eats smaller fish, and humans eat fish. The concentration of mercury in humans has now risen. Biomagnification is affected by the persistence of a chemical, whether it can be broken down and negated, food chain energetics, and whether organisms can reduce or negate the substance.

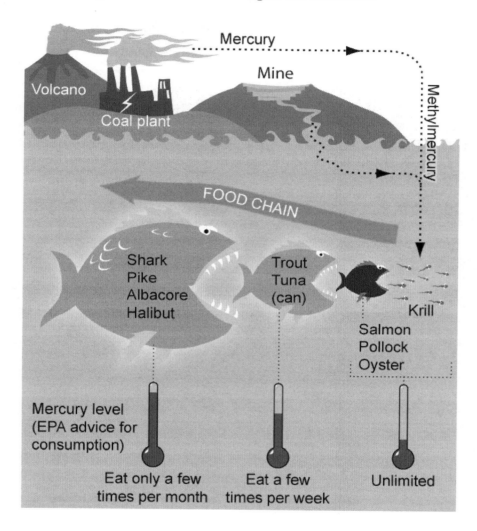

A food web consists of interconnected food chains in a community. The organisms can be linked to show the direction of energy flow. Energy flow in this sense is used to refer to the actual caloric flow through a system from trophic level to trophic level. Trophic level refers to a link in a food chain or a level of nutrition. The 10% rule is that from trophic level to level, about 90% of the energy is lost (in the form of heat, for example). The lowest trophic level consists of primary producers (usually plants), then primary consumers, then secondary consumers, and finally tertiary consumers (large carnivores). The final link is decomposers, which break down the consumers at the top. Food chains usually do not contain more than six links. These links may also be referred to as ecological pyramids.

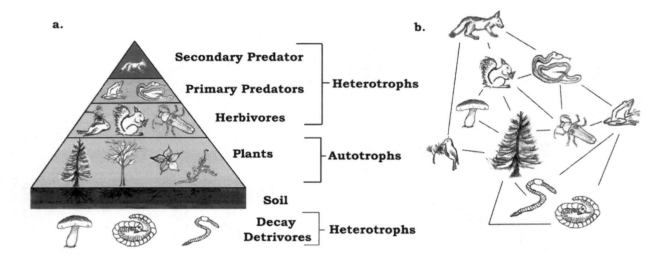

Ecosystem stability is a concept that states that a stable ecosystem is perfectly efficient. Seasonal changes or expected climate fluctuations are balanced by homeostasis. It also states that interspecies interactions are part of the balance of the system. Four principles of ecosystem stability are that waste disposal and nutrient replenishment by recycling is complete, the system uses sunlight as an energy source, biodiversity remains, and populations are stable in that they do not over consume resources. Ecologic succession is the concept that states that there is an orderly progression of change within a community. An example of primary succession is that over hundreds of years bare rock decomposes to sand, which eventually leads to soil formation, which eventually leads to the growth of grasses and trees. Secondary succession occurs after a disturbance or major event that greatly affects a community, such as a wild fire or construction of a dam.

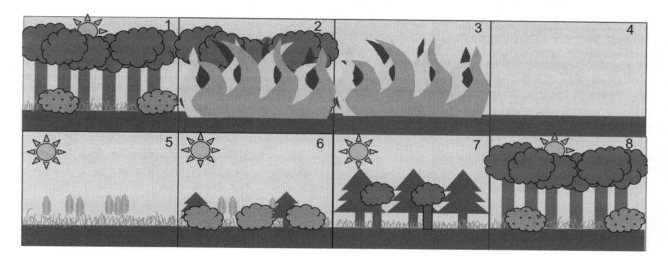

Population is a measure of how many individuals exist in a specific area. It can be used to measure the size of human, plant, or animal groups. Population growth depends on many factors. Factors that can limit the number of individuals in a population include lack of resources such as food and water, space, habitat destruction, competition, disease, and predators. Exponential growth refers to an unlimited rising growth rate. This kind of growth can be plotted on a chart in the shape of a J. Carrying capacity is the population size that can be sustained. The world's population is about 6.8 billion and growing. The human population has not yet reached its carrying capacity. Population dynamics refers to how a population changes over time and the factors that cause changes. An S-shaped curve shows that population growth has leveled off. Biotic potential refers to the maximum reproductive capacity of a population given ideal environmental conditions.

Biological concepts:

Territoriality: This refers to members of a species protecting areas from other members of their species and from other species. Species members claim specific areas as their own.

Dominance: This refers to the species in a community that is the most populous.

Altruism: This is when a species or individual in a community exhibits behaviors that benefit another individual at a cost to itself. In biology, altruism does not have to be a conscious sacrifice.

Threat display: This refers to behavior by an organism that is intended to intimidate or frighten away members of its own or another species.

The principle of **competitive exclusion** (Gause's Law) states that if there are limited or insufficient resources and species are competing for them, these species will not be able to co-exist. The result is that one of the species will become extinct or be forced to undergo a behavioral or evolutionary change. Another way to say this is that "complete competitors cannot coexist."

A **community** is any number of species interacting within a given area. A **niche** is the role of a species within a community. **Species diversity** refers to the number of species within a community and their populations. A **biome** refers to an area in which species are associated because of climate. The six major biomes in North America are desert, tropical rain forest, grassland, coniferous forest, deciduous forest, and tundra.

Biotic: Biotic factors are the living factors, such as other organisms, that affect a community or population. Abiotic factors are nonliving factors that affect a community or population, such as facets of the environment.

Ecology: Ecology is the study of plants, animals, their environments, and how they interact.

Ecosystem: An ecosystem is a community of species and all of the environment factors that affect them.

Biomass: In ecology, biomass refers to the mass of one or all of the species (species biomass) in an ecosystem or area.

Predation, parasitism, commensalism, and mutualism are all types of species interactions that affect species populations. **Intraspecific relationships** are relationships among members of a species. **Interspecific relationships** are relationships between members of different species.

Predation: This is a relationship in which one individual feeds on another (the prey), causing the prey to die. **Mimicry** is an adaptation developed as a response to predation. It refers to an organism that has a similar appearance to another species, which is meant to fool the predator into thinking the organism is more dangerous than it really is. Two examples are the drone fly and the io moth. The fly looks like a bee, but cannot sting. The io moth has markings on its wings that make it look like an owl. The moth can startle predators and gain time to escape. Predators can also use mimicry to lure their prey.

Commensalism: This refers to interspecific relationships in which one of the organisms benefits.

Mutualism, competition, and parasitism are all types of commensalism.

Mutualism: This is a relationship in which both organisms benefit from an interaction.
Competition: This is a relationship in which both organisms are harmed.
Parasitism: This is a relationship in which one organism benefits and the other is harmed.

Chemistry

Atoms

Matter refers to substances that have mass and occupy space (or volume). The traditional definition of matter describes it as having three states: solid, liquid, and gas. These different states are caused by differences in the distances and angles between molecules or atoms, which result in differences in the energy that binds them. Solid structures are rigid or nearly rigid and have strong bonds. Molecules or atoms of liquids move around and have weak bonds, although they are not weak enough to readily break. Molecules or atoms of gases move almost independently of each other, are typically far apart, and do not form bonds. The current definition of matter describes it as having four states. The fourth is plasma, which is an ionized gas that has some electrons that are described as free because they are not bound to an atom or molecule.

All matter consists of atoms. Atoms consist of a nucleus and electrons. The nucleus consists of protons and neutrons. The properties of these are measurable; they have mass and an electrical charge. The nucleus is positively charged due to the presence of protons. Electrons are negatively charged and orbit the nucleus. The nucleus has considerably more mass than the surrounding electrons. Atoms can bond together to make molecules. Atoms that have an equal number of protons and electrons are electrically neutral. If the number of protons and electrons in an atom is not equal, the atom has a positive or negative charge and is an ion.

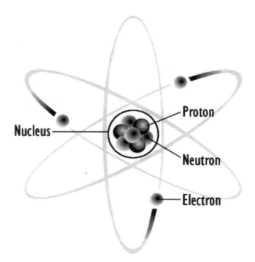

An element is matter with one particular type of atom. It can be identified by its atomic number, or the number of protons in its nucleus. There are approximately 117 elements currently known, 94 of which occur naturally on Earth. Elements from the periodic table include hydrogen, carbon, iron, helium, mercury, and oxygen. Atoms combine to form molecules. For example, two atoms of hydrogen (H) and one atom of oxygen (O) combine to form water (H_2O).

Compounds are substances containing two or more elements. Compounds are formed by chemical reactions and frequently have different properties than the original elements. Compounds are

- 66 -

decomposed by a chemical reaction rather than separated by a physical one. Solutions are homogeneous mixtures composed of two or more substances that have become one. Mixtures contain two or more substances that are combined but have not reacted chemically with each other. Mixtures can be separated using physical methods, while compounds cannot.

A solution is a homogeneous mixture. A mixture is two or more different substances that are mixed together, but not combined chemically. Homogeneous mixtures are those that are uniform in their composition. Solutions consist of a solute (the substance that is dissolved) and a solvent (the substance that does the dissolving). An example is sugar water. The solvent is the water and the solute is the sugar. The intermolecular attraction between the solvent and the solute is called solvation. Hydration refers to solutions in which water is the solvent. Solutions are formed when the forces of the molecules of the solute and the solvent are as strong as the individual molecular forces of the solute and the solvent. An example is that salt ($NaCl$) dissolves in water to create a solution. The Na^+ and the Cl^- ions in salt interact with the molecules of water and vice versa to overcome the individual molecular forces of the solute and the solvent.

Elements are represented in upper case letters. If there is no subscript, it indicates there is only one atom of the element. Otherwise, the subscript indicates the number of atoms. In molecular formulas, elements are organized according to the Hill system. Carbon is first, hydrogen comes next, and the remaining elements are listed in alphabetical order. If there is no carbon, all elements are listed alphabetically. There are a couple of exceptions to these rules. First, oxygen is usually listed last in oxides. Second, in ionic compounds the positive ion is listed first, followed by the negative ion. In CO_2, for example, C indicates 1 atom of carbon and O_2 indicates 2 atoms of oxygen. The compound is carbon dioxide. The formula for ammonia (an ionic compound) is NH_3, which is one atom of nitrogen and three of hydrogen. H_2O is two atoms of hydrogen and one of oxygen. Sugar is $C_6H_{12}O_6$, which is 6 atoms of carbon, 12 of hydrogen, and 6 of oxygen.

An **atom** is one of the most basic units of matter. An atom consists of a central nucleus surrounded by electrons. The **nucleus** of an atom consists of protons and neutrons. It is positively charged, dense, and heavier than the surrounding electrons. The plural form of nucleus is nuclei. **Neutrons** are the uncharged atomic particles contained within the nucleus. The number of neutrons in a nucleus can be represented as "N." Along with neutrons, **protons** make up the nucleus of an atom. The number of protons in the nucleus determines the atomic number of an element. Carbon atoms, for example, have six protons. The atomic number of carbon is 6. **Nucleon** refers collectively to neutrons and protons. **Electrons** are atomic particles that are negatively charged and orbit the nucleus of an atom. The number of protons minus the number of electrons indicates the charge of an atom.

The **atomic number** of an element refers to the number of protons in the nucleus of an atom. It is a unique identifier. It can be represented as Z. Atoms with a neutral charge have an atomic number that is equal to the number of electrons. **Atomic mass** is also known as the mass number. The atomic mass is the total number of protons and neutrons in the nucleus of an atom. It is referred to as "A." The atomic mass (A) is equal to the number of protons (Z) plus the number of neutrons (N).

This can be represented by the equation A = Z + N. The mass of electrons in an atom is basically insignificant because it is so small. **Atomic weight** may sometimes be referred to as "relative atomic mass," but should not be confused with atomic mass. Atomic weight is the ratio of the average mass per atom of a sample (which can include various isotopes of an element) to 1/12 of the mass of an atom of carbon-12.

Chemical properties are qualities of a substance which can't be determined by simply looking at the substance and must be determined through chemical reactions. Some chemical properties of elements include: atomic number, electron configuration, electrons per shell, electronegativity, atomic radius, and isotopes.

In contrast to chemical properties, **physical properties** can be observed or measured without chemical reactions. These include properties such as color, elasticity, mass, volume, and temperature. **Mass** is a measure of the amount of substance in an object. **Weight** is a measure of the gravitational pull of Earth on an object. **Volume** is a measure of the amount of space occupied. There are many formulas to determine volume. For example, the volume of a cube is the length of one side cubed (a^3) and the volume of a rectangular prism is length times width times height ($l \cdot w \cdot h$). The volume of an irregular shape can be determined by how much water it displaces. **Density** is a measure of the amount of mass per unit volume. The formula to find density is mass divided by volume ($D = m/V$). It is expressed in terms of mass per cubic unit, such as grams per cubic centimeter (g/cm^3). **Specific gravity** is a measure of the ratio of a substance's density compared to the density of water.

> ➢ **Review Video: <u>Mass, Weight, Volume, Density, and Specific Gravity</u>**
> *Visit **mometrix.com/academy** and enter **Code: 920570***

Both physical changes and chemical reactions are everyday occurrences. Physical changes do not result in different substances. For example, when water becomes ice it has undergone a physical change, but not a chemical change. It has changed its form, but not its composition. It is still H_2O. Chemical properties are concerned with the constituent particles that make up the physicality of a substance. Chemical properties are apparent when chemical changes occur. The chemical properties of a substance are influenced by its electron configuration, which is determined in part by the number of protons in the nucleus (the atomic number). Carbon, for example, has 6 protons and 6 electrons. It is an element's outermost valence electrons that mainly determine its chemical properties. Chemical reactions may release or consume energy.

Periodic Table

The periodic table groups elements with similar chemical properties together. The grouping of elements is based on atomic structure. It shows periodic trends of physical and chemical properties and identifies families of elements with similar properties. It is a common model for organizing and understanding elements. In the periodic table, each element has its own cell that includes varying amounts of information presented in symbol form about the properties of the element. Cells in the table are arranged in rows (periods) and columns (groups or families). At minimum, a cell includes the symbol for the element and its atomic number. The cell for hydrogen, for example, which appears first in the upper left corner, includes an "H" and a "1" above the letter. Elements are ordered by atomic number, left to right, top to bottom.

➢ **Review Video: Periodic Table**
*Visit **mometrix.com/academy** and enter **Code: 154828***

In the periodic table, the groups are the columns numbered 1 through 18 that group elements with similar outer electron shell configurations. Since the configuration of the outer electron shell is one of the primary factors affecting an element's chemical properties, elements within the same group have similar chemical properties. Previous naming conventions for groups have included the use of Roman numerals and upper-case letters. Currently, the periodic table groups are: Group 1, alkali metals; Group 2, alkaline earth metals; Groups 3-12, transition metals; Group 13, boron family; Group 14; carbon family; Group 15, pnictogens; Group 16, chalcogens; Group 17, halogens; Group 18, noble gases.

In the periodic table, there are seven periods (rows), and within each period there are blocks that group elements with the same outer electron subshell (more on this in the next section). The number of electrons in that outer shell determines which group an element belongs to within a given block. Each row's number (1, 2, 3, etc.) corresponds to the highest number electron shell that is in use. For example, row 2 uses only electron shells 1 and 2, while row 7 uses all shells from 1-7.

Atomic radii will decrease from left to right across a period (row) on the periodic table. In a group (column), there is an increase in the atomic radii of elements from top to bottom. Ionic radii will be smaller than the atomic radii for metals, but the opposite is true for non-metals. From left to right, electronegativity, or an atom's likeliness of taking another atom's electrons, increases. In a group, electronegativity decreases from top to bottom. Ionization energy or the amount of energy needed to get rid of an atom's outermost electron, increases across a period and decreases down a group. Electron affinity will become more negative across a period but will not change much within a group. The melting point decreases from top to bottom in the metal groups and increases from top to bottom in the non-metal groups.

Group→	1	2	3	4	5	6	7	8	9	10	11	12	13	14	15	16	17	18
↓Period																		
1	1 H																	2 He
2	3 Li	4 Be											5 B	6 C	7 N	8 O	9 F	10 Ne
3	11 Na	12 Mg											13 Al	14 Si	15 P	16 S	17 Cl	18 Ar
4	19 K	20 Ca	21 Sc	22 Ti	23 V	24 Cr	25 Mn	26 Fe	27 Co	28 Ni	29 Cu	30 Zn	31 Ga	32 Ge	33 As	34 Se	35 Br	36 Kr
5	37 Rb	38 Sr	39 Y	40 Zr	41 Nb	42 Mo	43 Tc	44 Ru	45 Rh	46 Pd	47 Ag	48 Cd	49 In	50 Sn	51 Sb	52 Te	53 I	54 Xe
6	55 Cs	56 Ba	*	72 Hf	73 Ta	74 W	75 Re	76 Os	77 Ir	78 Pt	79 Au	80 Hg	81 Tl	82 Pb	83 Bi	84 Po	85 At	86 Rn
7	87 Fr	88 Ra	**	104 Rf	105 Db	106 Sg	107 Bh	108 Hs	109 Mt	110 Ds	111 Rg	112 Cn	113 Uut	114 Fl	115 Uup	116 Lv	117 Uus	118 Uuo

*	57 La	58 Ce	59 Pr	60 Nd	61 Pm	62 Sm	63 Eu	64 Gd	65 Tb	66 Dy	67 Ho	68 Er	69 Tm	70 Yb	71 Lu
**	89 Ac	90 Th	91 Pa	92 U	93 Np	94 Pu	95 Am	96 Cm	97 Bk	98 Cf	99 Es	100 Fm	101 Md	102 No	103 Lr

Electrons

Electrons are subatomic particles that orbit the nucleus at various levels commonly referred to as layers, shells, or clouds. The orbiting electron or electrons account for only a fraction of the atom's mass. They are much smaller than the nucleus, are negatively charged, and exhibit wave-like characteristics. Electrons are part of the lepton family of elementary particles. Electrons can occupy orbits that are varying distances away from the nucleus, and tend to occupy the lowest energy level they can. If an atom has all its electrons in the lowest available positions, it has a stable electron arrangement. The outermost electron shell of an atom in its uncombined state is known as the valence shell. The electrons there are called valence electrons, and it is their number that determines bonding behavior. Atoms tend to react in a manner that will allow them to fill or empty their valence shells.

There are seven electron shells. One is closest to the nucleus and seven is the farthest away. Electron shells can also be identified with the letters K, L, M, N, O, P, and Q. Traditionally, there were four subshells identified by the first letter of their descriptive name: s (sharp), p (principal), d (diffuse), and f (fundamental). The maximum number of electrons for each subshell is as follows: s is 2, p is 6, d is 10, and f is 14. Every shell has an s subshell, the second shell and those above also have a p subshell, the third shell and those above also have a d subshell, and so on. Each subshell contains atomic orbitals, which describes the wave-like characteristics of an electron or a pair of electrons expressed as two angles and the distance from the nucleus. Atomic orbital is a concept used to express the likelihood of an electron's position in accordance with the idea of wave-particle duality.

Electron configuration: This is a trend whereby electrons fill shells and subshells in an element in a particular order and with a particular number of electrons. The chemical properties of the elements reflect their electron configurations. Energy levels (shells) do not have to be completely filled before the next one begins to be filled. An example of electron configuration notation is $1s^22s^22p^5$, where the first number is the row (period), or shell. The letter refers to the subshell of the shell, and the number in superscript is the number of electrons in the subshell. A common shorthand method for electron configuration notation is to use a noble gas (in a bracket) to abbreviate the shells that elements have in common. For example, the electron configuration for neon is $1s^22s^22p^6$. The configuration for phosphorus is $1s^22s^22p^63s^23p^3$, which can be written as $[Ne]3s^23p^3$. Subshells are filled in the following manner: 1s, 2s, 2p, 3s, 3p, 4s, 3d, 4p, 5s, 4d, 5p, 6s, 4f, 5d, 6p, 7s, 5f, 6d, and 7p.

Most atoms are neutral since the positive charge of the protons in the nucleus is balanced by the negative charge of the surrounding electrons. Electrons are transferred between atoms when they come into contact with each other. This creates a molecule or atom in which the number of electrons does not equal the number of protons, which gives it a positive or negative charge. A negative ion is created when an atom gains electrons, while a positive ion is created when an atom loses electrons. An ionic bond is formed between ions with opposite charges. The resulting compound is neutral. Ionization refers to the process by which neutral particles are ionized into charged particles. Gases and plasmas can be partially or fully ionized through ionization.

Atoms interact by transferring or sharing the electrons furthest from the nucleus. Known as the outer or valence electrons, they are responsible for the chemical properties of an element. Bonds between atoms are created when electrons are paired up by being transferred or shared. If electrons are transferred from one atom to another, the bond is ionic. If electrons are shared, the bond is covalent. Atoms of the same element may bond together to form molecules or crystalline solids. When two or more different types of atoms bind together chemically, a compound is made. The physical properties of compounds reflect the nature of the interactions among their molecules. These interactions are determined by the structure of the molecule, including the atoms they consist of and the distances and angles between them.

Isotopes and Molecules

The number of protons in an atom determines the element of that atom. For instance, all helium atoms have exactly two protons, and all oxygen atoms have exactly eight protons. If two atoms have the same number of protons, then they are the same element. However, the number of neutrons in two atoms can be different without the atoms being different elements. Isotope is the term used to distinguish between atoms that have the same number of protons but a different number of neutrons. The names of isotopes have the element name with the mass number. Recall that the mass number is the number of protons plus the number of neutrons. For example, carbon-12 refers to an atom that has 6 protons, which makes it carbon, and 6 neutrons. In other words, 6 protons + 6 neutrons = 12. Carbon-13 has six protons and seven neutrons, and carbon-14 has six protons and eight neutrons. Isotopes can also be written with the mass number in superscript before the element symbol. For example, carbon-12 can be written as ^{12}C.

> ➤ **Review Video: Isotopes**
> *Visit mometrix.com/academy and enter Code: 294271*

The important properties of water (H_2O) are high polarity, hydrogen bonding, cohesiveness, adhesiveness, high specific heat, high latent heat, and high heat of vaporization. It is essential to life as we know it, as water is one of the main if not the main constituent of many living things. Water is a liquid at room temperature. The high specific heat of water means it resists the breaking of its hydrogen bonds and resists heat and motion, which is why it has a relatively high boiling point and high vaporization point. It also resists temperature change. Water is peculiar in that its solid state floats in its liquid state. Most substances are denser in their solid forms. Water is cohesive, which means it is attracted to itself. It is also adhesive, which means it readily attracts other molecules. If water tends to adhere to another substance, the substance is said to be hydrophilic. Water makes a good solvent. Substances, particularly those with polar ions and molecules, readily dissolve in water.

Electrons in an atom can orbit different levels around the nucleus. They can absorb or release energy, which can change the location of their orbit or even allow them to break free from the atom. The outermost layer is the valence layer, which contains the valence electrons. The valence layer tends to have or share eight electrons. Molecules are formed by a chemical bond between atoms, a bond which occurs at the valence level.

Two basic types of bonds are covalent and ionic. A covalent bond is formed when atoms share electrons. An ionic bond is formed when an atom transfers an electron to another atom. A hydrogen bond is a weak bond between a hydrogen atom of one molecule and an electronegative atom (such as nitrogen, oxygen, or fluorine) of another molecule. The Van der Waals force is a weak force between molecules. This type of force is much weaker than actual chemical bonds between atoms.

Reactions

Chemical reactions measured in human time can take place quickly or slowly. They can take fractions of a second or billions of years. The rates of chemical reactions are determined by how frequently reacting atoms and molecules interact. Rates are also influenced by the temperature and various properties (such as shape) of the reacting materials. Catalysts accelerate chemical reactions, while inhibitors decrease reaction rates. Some types of reactions release energy in the form of heat and light. Some types of reactions involve the transfer of either electrons or hydrogen ions between reacting ions, molecules, or atoms. In other reactions, chemical bonds are broken down by heat or light to form reactive radicals with electrons that will readily form new bonds. Processes such as the formation of ozone and greenhouse gases in the atmosphere and the burning and processing of fossil fuels are controlled by radical reactions.

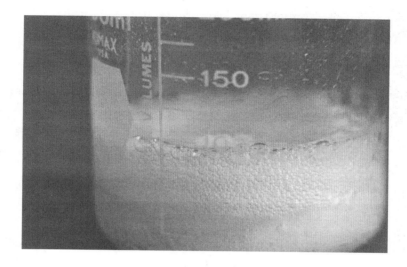

Chemical equations describe chemical reactions. The reactants are on the left side before the arrow and the products are on the right side after the arrow. The arrow indicates the reaction or change. The coefficient, or stoichiometric coefficient, is the number before the element, and indicates the ratio of reactants to products in terms of moles. The equation for the formation of water from hydrogen and oxygen, for example, is $2H_{2(g)} + O_{2(g)} \rightarrow 2H_2O_{(l)}$. The 2 preceding hydrogen and water is the coefficient, which means there are 2 moles of hydrogen and 2 of water. There is 1 mole of oxygen, which does not have to be indicated with the number 1. In parentheses, g stands for gas, l stands for liquid, s stands for solid, and aq stands for aqueous solution (a substance dissolved in water). Charges are shown in superscript for individual ions, but not for ionic compounds. Polyatomic ions are separated by parentheses so the ion will not be confused with the number of ions.

An unbalanced equation is one that does not follow the law of conservation of mass, which states that matter can only be changed, not created. If an equation is unbalanced, the numbers of atoms indicated by the stoichiometric coefficients on each side of the arrow will not be equal. Start by writing the formulas for each species in the reaction. Count the atoms on each side and determine if the number is equal. Coefficients must be whole numbers. Fractional amounts, such as half a molecule, are not possible. Equations can be balanced by multiplying the coefficients by a constant that will produce the smallest possible whole number coefficient. $H_2 + O_2 \rightarrow H_2O$ is an example of an unbalanced equation. The balanced equation is $2H_2 + O_2 \rightarrow 2H_2O$, which indicates that it takes two moles of hydrogen and one of oxygen to produce two moles of water.

One way to organize chemical reactions is to sort them into two categories: oxidation/reduction reactions (also called redox reactions) and metathesis reactions (which include acid/base reactions). Oxidation/reduction reactions can involve the transfer of one or more electrons, or they can occur as a result of the transfer of oxygen, hydrogen, or halogen atoms. The species that loses electrons is oxidized and is referred to as the reducing agent. The species that gains electrons is reduced and is referred to as the oxidizing agent. The element undergoing oxidation experiences an increase in its oxidation number, while the element undergoing reduction experiences a decrease in its oxidation number. Single replacement reactions are types of oxidation/reduction reactions. In a single replacement reaction, electrons are transferred from one chemical species to another. The transfer of electrons results in changes in the nature and charge of the species.

Single substitution, displacement, or replacement reactions are when one reactant is displaced by another to form the final product ($A + BC \rightarrow B + AC$). Single substitution reactions can be cationic or anionic. When a piece of copper (Cu) is placed into a solution of silver nitrate ($AgNO_3$), the solution turns blue. The copper appears to be replaced with a silvery-white material. The equation is $2AgNO_3 + Cu \rightarrow Cu(NO_3)2 + 2Ag$. When this reaction takes place, the copper dissolves and the silver in the silver nitrate solution precipitates (becomes a solid), thus resulting in copper nitrate and silver. Copper and silver have switched places in the nitrate.

Combination, or synthesis, reactions: In a combination reaction, two or more reactants combine to form a single product ($A + B \rightarrow C$). These reactions are also called synthesis or addition reactions. An example is burning hydrogen in air to produce water. The equation is $2H_2\,_{(g)} + O_2\,_{(g)} \rightarrow 2H_2O\,_{(l)}$. Another example is when water and sulfur trioxide react to form sulfuric acid. The equation is $H_2O + SO_3 \rightarrow H_2SO_4$.

Double displacement, double replacement, substitution, metathesis, or ion exchange reactions are when ions or bonds are exchanged by two compounds to form different compounds ($AC + BD \rightarrow AD + BC$). An example of this is that silver nitrate and sodium chloride form two different products (silver chloride and sodium nitrate) when they react. The formula for this reaction is $AgNO_3 + NaCl \rightarrow AgCl + NaNO_3$.

Double replacement reactions are metathesis reactions. In a double replacement reaction, the chemical reactants exchange ions but the oxidation state stays the same. One of the indicators of this is the formation of a solid precipitate. In acid/base reactions, an acid is a compound that can donate a proton, while a base is a compound that can accept a proton. In these types of reactions, the acid and base react to form a salt and water. When the proton is donated, the base becomes water and the remaining ions form a salt. One method of determining whether a reaction is an oxidation/reduction or a metathesis reaction is that the oxidation number of atoms does not change during a metathesis reaction.

A neutralization, acid-base, or proton transfer reaction is when one compound acquires H^+ from another. These types of reactions are also usually double displacement reactions. The acid has an H^+ that is transferred to the base and neutralized to form a salt.

Decomposition (or desynthesis, decombination, or deconstruction) reactions; in a decomposition reaction, a reactant is broken down into two or more products ($A \rightarrow B + C$). These reactions are also called analysis reactions. Thermal decomposition is caused by heat. Electrolytic decomposition is due to electricity. An example of this type of reaction is the decomposition of water into hydrogen and oxygen gas. The equation is $2H_2O \rightarrow 2H_2 + O_2$. Decomposition is considered a chemical reaction whereby a single compound breaks down into component parts or simpler compounds. When a compound or substance separates into these simpler substances, the byproducts are often substances that are different from the original. Decomposition can be viewed as the opposite of combination reactions. Most decomposition reactions are endothermic. Heat needs to be added for the chemical reaction to occur. Separation processes can be mechanical or chemical, and usually involve re-organizing a mixture of substances without changing their chemical nature. The separated products may differ from the original mixture in terms of chemical or physical properties. Types of separation processes include filtration, crystallization, distillation, and chromatography. Basically, decomposition breaks down one compound into two or more compounds or substances that are different from the original; separation sorts the substances from the original mixture into like substances.

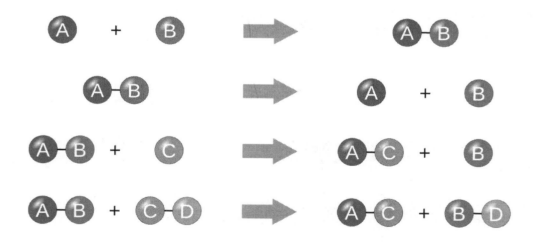

Endothermic reactions are chemical reactions that absorb heat and exothermic reactions are chemical reactions that release heat. Reactants are the substances that are consumed during a reaction, while products are the substances that are produced or formed. A balanced equation is one that uses reactants, products, and coefficients in such a way that the number of each type of atom (law of conservation of mass) and the total charge remains the same. The reactants are on the left side of the arrow and the products are on the right. The heat difference between endothermic and exothermic reactions is caused by bonds forming and breaking. If more energy is needed to break the reactant bonds than is released when they form, the reaction is endothermic. Heat is absorbed and the environmental temperature decreases. If more energy is released when product bonds form than is needed to break the reactant bonds, the reaction is exothermic. Heat is released and the environmental temperature increases.

The collision theory states that for a chemical reaction to occur, atoms or molecules have to collide with each other with a certain amount of energy. A certain amount of energy is required to breach the activation barrier. Heating a mixture will raise the energy levels of the molecules and the rate of reaction (the time it takes for a reaction to complete). Generally, the rate of reaction is doubled for every 10 degrees Celsius temperature increase. However, the increase needed to double a reaction rate increases as the temperature climbs. This is due to the increase in collision frequency that occurs as the temperature increases. Other factors that can affect the rate of reaction are surface area, concentration, pressure, and the presence of a catalyst.

The particles of an atom's nucleus (the protons and neutrons) are bound together by nuclear force, also known as residual strong force. Unlike chemical reactions, which involve electrons, nuclear reactions occur when two nuclei or nuclear particles collide. This results in the release or absorption of energy and products that are different from the initial particles. The energy released in a nuclear reaction can take various forms, including the release of kinetic energy of the product particles and the emission of very high energy photons known as gamma rays. Some energy may also remain in the nucleus. Radioactivity refers to the particles emitted from nuclei as a result of nuclear instability. There are many nuclear isotopes that are unstable and can spontaneously emit some kind of radiation. The most common types of radiation are alpha, beta, and gamma radiation, but there are several other varieties of radioactive decay.

Inorganic and Organic

The terms inorganic and organic have become less useful over time as their definitions have changed. Historically, inorganic molecules were defined as those of a mineral nature that were not created by biological processes. Organic molecules were defined as those that were produced biologically by a "life process" or "vital force." It was then discovered that organic compounds could be synthesized without a life process.

Currently, molecules containing carbon are considered organic. Carbon is largely responsible for creating biological diversity, and is more capable than all other elements of forming large, complex, and diverse molecules of an organic nature. Carbon often completes its valence shell by sharing electrons with other atoms in four covalent bonds, which is also known as tetravalence.

The main trait of inorganic compounds is that they lack carbon. Inorganic compounds include mineral salts, metals and alloys, non-metallic compounds such as phosphorus, and metal complexes. A metal complex has a central atom (or ion) bonded to surrounding ligands (molecules or anions). The ligands sacrifice the donor atoms (in the form of at least one pair of electrons) to the central atom. Many inorganic compounds are ionic, meaning they form ionic bonds rather than share electrons. They may have high melting points because of this. They may also be colorful, but this is not an absolute identifier of an inorganic compound. Salts, which are inorganic compounds, are an example of inorganic bonding of cations and anions. Some examples of salts are magnesium chloride ($MgCl_2$) and sodium oxide (Na_2O). Oxides, carbonates, sulfates, and halides are classes of inorganic compounds. They are typically poor conductors, are very water soluble, and crystallize easily. Minerals and silicates are also inorganic compounds.

Two of the main characteristics of organic compounds are that they include carbon and are formed by covalent bonds. Carbon can form long chains, double and triple bonds, and rings. While inorganic compounds tend to have high melting points, organic compounds tend to melt at temperatures below 300° C. They also tend to boil, sublimate, and decompose below this temperature. Unlike inorganic compounds, they are not very water soluble. Organic molecules are organized into functional groups based on their specific atoms, which helps determine how they will react chemically. A few groups are alkanes, nitro, alkenes, sulfides, amines, and carbolic acids. The hydroxyl group (-OH) consists of alcohols. These molecules are polar, which increases their solubility. By some estimates, there are more than 16 million organic compounds.

Nomenclature refers to the manner in which a compound is named. First, it must be determined whether the compound is ionic (formed through electron transfer between cations and anions) or molecular (formed through electron sharing between molecules). When dealing with an ionic compound, the name is determined using the standard naming conventions for ionic compounds. This involves indicating the positive element first (the charge must be defined when there is more than one option for the valency) followed by the negative element plus the appropriate suffix. The rules for naming a molecular compound are as follows: write elements in order of increasing group number and determine the prefix by determining the number of atoms. Exclude mono for the first atom. The name for CO_2, for example, is carbon dioxide. The end of oxygen is dropped and "ide" is added to make oxide, and the prefix "di" is used to indicate there are two atoms of oxygen.

Acids and Bases

The potential of hydrogen (pH) is a measurement of the concentration of hydrogen ions in a substance in terms of the number of moles of H^+ per liter of solution. All substances fall between 0 and 14 on the pH scale. A lower pH indicates a higher H^+ concentration, while a higher pH indicates a lower H^+ concentration. Pure water has a neutral pH, which is 7. Anything with a pH lower than water (0-7) is considered acidic. Anything with a pH higher than water (7-14) is a base. Drain cleaner, soap, baking soda, ammonia, egg whites, and sea water are common bases. Urine, stomach acid, citric acid, vinegar, hydrochloric acid, and battery acid are acids. A pH indicator is a substance that acts as a detector of hydrogen or hydronium ions. It is halochromic, meaning it changes color to indicate that hydrogen or hydronium ions have been detected.

When they are dissolved in aqueous solutions, some properties of acids are that they conduct electricity, change blue litmus paper to red, have a sour taste, react with bases to neutralize them, and react with active metals to free hydrogen. A weak acid is one that does not donate all of its protons or disassociate completely. Strong acids include hydrochloric, hydriodic, hydrobromic, perchloric, nitric, and sulfuric. They ionize completely. Superacids are those that are stronger than 100 percent sulfuric acid. They include fluoroantimonic, magic, and perchloric acids. Acids can be used in pickling, a process used to remove rust and corrosion from metals. They are also used as catalysts in the processing of minerals and the production of salts and fertilizers. Phosphoric acid (H_3PO_4) is added to sodas and other acids are added to foods as preservatives or to add taste.

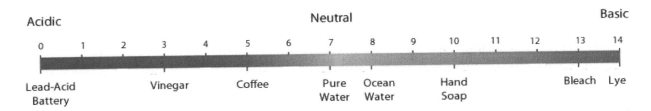

When they are dissolved in aqueous solutions, some properties of bases are that they conduct electricity, change red litmus paper to blue, feel slippery, and react with acids to neutralize their properties. A weak base is one that does not completely ionize in an aqueous solution, and usually has a low pH. Strong bases can free protons in very weak acids. Examples of strong bases are hydroxide compounds such as potassium, barium, and lithium hydroxides. Most are in the first and second groups of the periodic table. A superbase is extremely strong compared to sodium hydroxide and cannot be kept in an aqueous solution. Superbases are organized into organic, organometallic, and inorganic classes. Bases are used as insoluble catalysts in heterogeneous reactions and as catalysts in hydrogenation.

Some properties of salts are that they are formed from acid base reactions, are ionic compounds consisting of metallic and nonmetallic ions, dissociate in water, and are comprised of tightly bonded ions. Some common salts are sodium chloride (NaCl), sodium bisulfate, potassium dichromate ($K_2Cr_2O_7$), and calcium chloride ($CaCl_2$). Calcium chloride is used as a drying agent, and may be used to absorb moisture when freezing mixtures. Potassium nitrate (KNO_3) is used to make fertilizer and in the manufacture of explosives. Sodium nitrate ($NaNO_3$) is also used in the making of fertilizer. Baking soda (sodium bicarbonate) is a salt, as are Epsom salts [magnesium sulfate ($MgSO_4$)]. Salt and water can react to form a base and an acid. This is called a hydrolysis reaction.

A buffer is a solution whose pH remains relatively constant when a small amount of an acid or a base is added. It is usually made of a weak acid and its conjugate base (proton receiver) or one of its soluble salts. It can also be made of a weak base and its conjugate acid (proton donator) or one of its salts.

A constant pH is necessary in living cells because some living things can only live within a certain pH range. If that pH changes, the cells could die. Blood is an example of a buffer. A pKa is a measure of acid dissociation or the acid dissociation constant. Buffer solutions can help keep enzymes at the correct pH. They are also used in the fermentation process, in dyeing fabrics, and in the calibration of pH meters. An example of a buffer is HC_2H_3O (a weak acid) and $NaC_2H_3O_2$ (a salt containing the $C_2H_3O_2^-$ ion).

General Concepts

Lewis formulas: These show the bonding or nonbonding tendency of specific pairs of valence electrons. Lewis dot diagrams use dots to represent valence electrons. Dots are paired around an atom. When an atom forms a covalent bond with another atom, the elements share the dots as they would electrons. Double and triple bonds are indicated with additional adjacent dots. Methane (CH_4), for instance, would be shown as a C with 2 dots above, below, and to the right and left and an H next to each set of dots. In structural formulas, the dots are single lines.

Kekulé diagrams: Like Lewis dot diagrams, these are two-dimensional representations of chemical compounds. Covalent bonds are shown as lines between elements. Double and triple bonds are shown as two or three lines and unbonded valence electrons are shown as dots.

Molar mass: This refers to the mass of one mole of a substance (element or compound), usually measured in grams per mole (g/mol). This differs from molecular mass in that molecular mass is the mass of one molecule of a substance relative to the atomic mass unit (amu).

Atomic mass unit (amu) is the smallest unit of mass, and is equal to 1/12 of the mass of the carbon isotope carbon-12. A mole (mol) is a measurement of molecular weight that is equal to the molecule's amu in grams. For example, carbon has an amu of 12, so a mole of carbon weighs 12 grams. One mole is equal to about 6.0221415×10^{23} elementary entities, which are usually atoms or molecules. This amount is also known as the Avogadro constant or Avogadro's number (N_A). Another way to say this is that one mole of a substance is the same as one Avogadro's number of that substance. One mole of chlorine, for example, is 6.0221415×10^{23} chlorine atoms. The charge on one mole of electrons is referred to as a Faraday.

The kinetic theory of gases assumes that gas molecules are small compared to the distances between them and that they are in constant random motion. The attractive and repulsive forces between gas molecules are negligible. Their kinetic energy does not change with time as long as the temperature remains the same. The higher the temperature is, the greater the motion will be. As the temperature of a gas increases, so does the kinetic energy of the molecules. In other words, gas will occupy a greater volume as the temperature is increased and a lesser volume as the temperature is decreased. In addition, the same amount of gas will occupy a greater volume as the temperature increases, but pressure remains constant. At any given temperature, gas molecules have the same average kinetic energy. The ideal gas law is derived from the kinetic theory of gases.

Charles's law: This states that gases expand when they are heated. It is also known as the law of volumes.

> ➤ **Review Video: Charles's Law**
> *Visit **mometrix.com/academy** and enter **Code: 537776***

Boyle's law: This states that gases contract when pressure is applied to them. It also states that if temperature remains constant, the relationship between absolute pressure and volume is inversely proportional. When one increases, the other decreases. Considered a specialized case of the ideal gas law, Boyle's law is sometimes known as the Boyle-Mariotte law.

> ➤ **Review Video: Boyle's Law**
> *Visit **mometrix.com/academy** and enter **Code: 115757***

The ideal gas law is used to explain the properties of a gas under ideal pressure, volume, and temperature conditions. It is best suited for describing monatomic gases (gases in which atoms are not bound together) and gases at high temperatures and low pressures. It is not well-suited for instances in which a gas or its components are close to their condensation point. All collisions are perfectly elastic and there are no intermolecular attractive forces at work. The ideal gas law is a way to explain and measure the macroscopic properties of matter. It can be derived from the kinetic theory of gases, which deals with the microscopic properties of matter. The equation for the ideal gas law is PV = nRT, where "P" is absolute pressure, "V" is absolute volume, and "T" is absolute temperature. "R" refers to the universal gas constant, which is 8.3145 J/mol Kelvin, and "n" is the number of moles.

Physics

Thermodynamics

Thermodynamics is a branch of physics that studies the conversion of energy into work and heat. It is especially concerned with variables such as temperature, volume, and pressure. Thermodynamic equilibrium refers to objects that have the same temperature because heat is transferred between them to reach equilibrium. Thermodynamics takes places within three different types of systems; open, isolated, and closed systems. Open systems are capable of interacting with a surrounding environment and can exchange heat, work (energy), and matter outside their system boundaries. A closed system can exchange heat and work, but not matter. An isolated system cannot exchange heat, work, or matter with its surroundings. Its total energy and mass stay the same. In physics, surrounding environment refers to everything outside a thermodynamic system (system). The terms "surroundings" and "environment" are also used. The term "boundary" refers to the division between the system and its surroundings.

The laws of thermodynamics are generalized principles dealing with energy and heat.
- The zeroth law of thermodynamics states that two objects in thermodynamic equilibrium with a third object are also in equilibrium with each other. Being in thermodynamic equilibrium basically means that different objects are at the same temperature.
- The first law deals with conservation of energy. It states that neither mass nor energy can be destroyed; only converted from one form to another.

> ➤ **Review Video: <u>The First Law of Thermodynamics</u>**
> *Visit **mometrix.com/academy** and enter **Code: 340643***

- The second law states that the entropy (the amount of energy in a system that is no longer available for work or the amount of disorder in a system) of an isolated system can only increase. The second law also states that heat is not transferred from a lower-temperature system to a higher-temperature one unless additional work is done.

> ➤ **Review Video: <u>The Second Law of Thermodynamics</u>**
> *Visit **mometrix.com/academy** and enter **Code: 251848***

- The third law of thermodynamics states that as temperature approaches absolute zero, entropy approaches a constant minimum. It also states that a system cannot be cooled to absolute zero.

Thermal contact refers to energy transferred to a body by a means other than work. A system in thermal contact with another can exchange energy with it through the process of heat transfer. Thermal contact does not necessarily involve direct physical contact. Heat is energy that can be transferred from one body or system to another without work being done. Everything tends to become less organized and less useful over time (entropy). In all energy transfers, therefore, the overall result is that the heat is spread out so that objects are in thermodynamic equilibrium and the heat can no longer be transferred without additional work.

The laws of thermodynamics state that energy can be exchanged between physical systems as heat or work, and that systems are affected by their surroundings. It can be said that the total amount of energy in the universe is constant. The first law is mainly concerned with the conservation of energy and related concepts, which include the statement that energy can only be transferred or converted, not created or destroyed. The formula used to represent the first law is $\Delta U = Q - W$, where ΔU is the change in total internal energy of a system, Q is the heat added to the system, and W is the work done by the system. Energy can be transferred by conduction, convection, radiation, mass transfer, and other processes such as collisions in chemical and nuclear reactions. As transfers occur, the matter involved becomes less ordered and less useful. This tendency towards disorder is also referred to as entropy.

The second law of thermodynamics explains how energy can be used. In particular, it states that heat will not transfer spontaneously from a cold object to a hot object. Another way to say this is that heat transfers occur from higher temperatures to lower temperatures. Also covered under this law is the concept that systems not under the influence of external forces tend to become more disordered over time. This type of disorder can be expressed in terms of entropy.

Another principle covered under this law is that it is impossible to make a heat engine that can extract heat and convert it all to useful work. A thermal bottleneck occurs in machines that convert energy to heat and then use it to do work. These types of machines are less efficient than ones that are solely mechanical.

Conduction is a form of heat transfer that occurs at the molecular level. It is the result of molecular agitation that occurs within an object, body, or material while the material stays motionless. An example of this is when a frying pan is placed on a hot burner. At first, the handle is not hot. As the pan becomes hotter due to conduction, the handle eventually gets hot too. In this example, energy is being transferred down the handle toward the colder end because the higher speed particles collide with and transfer energy to the slower ones. When this happens, the original material becomes cooler and the second material becomes hotter until equilibrium is reached. Thermal conduction can also occur between two substances such as a cup of hot coffee and the colder surface it is placed on. Heat is transferred, but matter is not.

Convection refers to heat transfer that occurs through the movement or circulation of fluids (liquids or gases). Some of the fluid becomes or is hotter than the surrounding fluid, and is less dense. Heat is transferred away from the source of the heat to a cooler, denser area. Examples of convection are boiling water and the movement of warm and cold air currents in the atmosphere and the ocean. Forced convection occurs in convection ovens, where a fan helps circulate hot air.

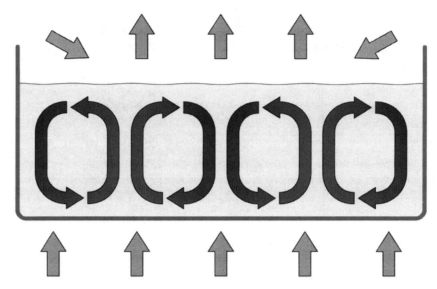

Radiation is heat transfer that occurs through the emission of electromagnetic waves, which carry energy away from the emitting object. All objects with temperatures above absolute zero radiate heat.

Temperature is a measurement of an object's stored heat energy. More specifically, temperature is the average kinetic energy of an object's particles. When the temperature of an object increases and its atoms move faster, kinetic energy also increases. Temperature is not energy since it changes and is not conserved. Thermometers are used to measure temperature.

There are three main scales for measuring temperature. Celsius uses the base reference points of water freezing at 0 degrees and boiling at 100 degrees. Fahrenheit uses the base reference points of water freezing at 32 degrees and boiling at 212 degrees. Celsius and Fahrenheit are both relative temperature scales since they use water as their reference point. The Kelvin temperature scale is an absolute temperature scale. Its zero mark corresponds to absolute zero. Water's freezing and boiling points are 273.15 Kelvin and 373.15 Kelvin, respectively. Where Celsius and Fahrenheit are measured is degrees, Kelvin does not use degree terminology.

- Converting Celsius to Fahrenheit: $°F = \frac{9}{5}°C + 32$
- Converting Fahrenheit to Celsius: $°C = \frac{5}{9}(°F - 32)$
- Converting Celsius to Kelvin: $K = °C + 273.15$
- Converting Kelvin to Celsius: $°C = K - 273.15$

Heat capacity, also known as thermal mass, refers to the amount of heat energy required to raise the temperature of an object, and is measured in Joules per Kelvin or Joules per degree Celsius. The equation for relating heat energy to heat capacity is $Q = C\Delta T$, where Q is the heat energy transferred, C is the heat capacity of the body, and ΔT is the change in the object's temperature. Specific heat capacity, also known as specific heat, is the heat capacity per unit mass. Every element and compound has its own specific heat. For example, it takes different amounts of heat energy to raise the temperature of the same amounts of magnesium and lead by one degree. The equation for relating heat energy to specific heat capacity is $Q = mc\Delta T$, where m represents the mass of the object, and c represents its specific heat capacity.

Some discussions of energy consider only two types of energy: kinetic energy (the energy of motion) and potential energy (which depends on relative position or orientation). There are, however, other types of energy. Electromagnetic waves, for example, are a type of energy contained by a field. Another type of potential energy is electrical energy, which is the energy it takes to pull apart positive and negative electrical charges. Chemical energy refers to the manner in which atoms form into molecules, and this energy can be released or absorbed when molecules regroup. Solar energy comes in the form of visible light and non-visible light, such as infrared and ultraviolet rays. Sound energy refers to the energy in sound waves.

Energy is constantly changing forms and being transferred back and forth. An example of a heat to mechanical energy transformation is a steam engine, such as the type used on a steam locomotive. A heat source such as coal is used to boil water. The steam produced turns a shaft, which eventually turns the wheels. A pendulum swinging is an example of both a kinetic to potential and a potential to kinetic energy transformation. When a pendulum is moved from its center point (the point at which it is closest to the ground) to the highest point before it returns, it is an example of a kinetic to potential transformation. When it swings from its highest point toward the center, it is considered a potential to kinetic transformation. The sum of the potential and kinetic energy is known as the total mechanical energy. Stretching a rubber band gives it potential energy. That potential energy becomes kinetic energy when the rubber band is released.

Motion and Force

Mechanics is the study of matter and motion, and the topics related to matter and motion, such as force, energy, and work. Discussions of mechanics will often include the concepts of vectors and scalars. Vectors are quantities with both magnitude and direction, while scalars have only magnitude. Scalar quantities include length, area, volume, mass, density, energy, work, and power. Vector quantities include displacement, direction, velocity, acceleration, momentum, and force.

Motion is a change in the location of an object, and is the result of an unbalanced net force acting on the object. Understanding motion requires the understanding of three basic quantities: displacement, velocity, and acceleration.

Displacement

When something moves from one place to another, it has undergone *displacement*. Displacement along a straight line is a very simple example of a vector quantity. If an object travels from position x = -5 cm to x = 5 cm, it has undergone a displacement of 10 cm. If it traverses the same path in the opposite direction, its displacement is -10 cm. A vector that spans the object's displacement in the direction of travel is known as a displacement vector.

> ➤ **Review Video: Displacement**
> *Visit mometrix.com/academy and enter Code:* **236197**

Velocity

There are two types of velocity to consider: *average velocity* and *instantaneous velocity*. Unless an object has a constant velocity or we are explicitly given an equation for the velocity, finding the instantaneous velocity of an object requires the use of calculus. If we want to calculate the *average velocity* of an object, we need to know two things: the displacement, or the distance it has covered, and the time it took to cover this distance. The formula for average velocity is simply the distance traveled divided by the time required. In other words, the average velocity is equal to the change in position divided by the change in time. Average velocity is a vector and will always point in the same direction as the displacement vector (since time is a scalar and always positive).

Acceleration

Acceleration is the change in the velocity of an object. On most test questions, the acceleration will be a constant value. Like position and velocity, acceleration is a vector quantity and will therefore have both magnitude and direction.

> ➤ **Review Video: Velocity and Acceleration**
> *Visit mometrix.com/academy and enter Code:* **671849**

Most motion can be explained by Newton's three laws of motion:

Newton's first law

An object at rest or in motion will remain at rest or in motion unless acted upon by an external force. This phenomenon is commonly referred to as inertia, the tendency of a body to remain in its present state of motion. In order for the body's state of motion to change, it must be acted on by an unbalanced force.

> ➤ **Review Video: Newton's First Law of Motion**
> *Visit mometrix.com/academy and enter Code:* **590367**

Newton's second law

An object's acceleration is directly proportional to the net force acting on the object, and inversely proportional to the object's mass. It is generally written in equation form $F = ma$, where F is the net force acting on a body, m is the mass of the body, and a is its acceleration. Note that since the mass is always a positive quantity, the acceleration is always in the same direction as the force.

> ➤ **Review Video: Newton's Second Law of Motion**
> *Visit **mometrix.com/academy** and enter **Code: 737975***

Newton's third law

For every force, there is an equal and opposite force. When a hammer strikes a nail, the nail hits the hammer just as hard. If we consider two objects, A and B, then we may express any contact between these two bodies with the equation $F_{AB} = -F_{BA}$, where the order of the subscripts denotes which body is exerting the force.

At first glance, this law might seem to forbid any movement at all since every force is being countered with an equal opposite force, but these equal opposite forces are acting on different bodies with different masses, so they will not cancel each other out.

> ➤ **Review Video: Newton's Third Law of Motion**
> *Visit **mometrix.com/academy** and enter **Code: 838401***

Energy

The two types of energy most important in mechanics are potential and kinetic energy. Potential energy is the amount of energy an object has stored within itself because of its position or orientation. There are many types of potential energy, but the most common is gravitational potential energy. It is the energy that an object has because of its height (h) above the ground. It can be calculated as $PE = mgh$, where m is the object's mass and g is the acceleration of gravity. Kinetic energy is the energy of an object in motion, and is calculated as $KE = mv^2/2$, where v is the magnitude of its velocity. When an object is dropped, its potential energy is converted into kinetic energy as it falls. These two equations can be used to calculate the velocity of an object at any point in its fall.

> ➤ **Review Video: Potential and Kinetic Energy**
> *Visit **mometrix.com/academy** and enter **Code: 491502***

Work

Work can be thought of as the amount of energy expended in accomplishing some goal. The simplest equation for mechanical work (W) is $W = Fd$, where F is the force exerted and d is the displacement of the object on which the force is exerted. This equation requires that the force be applied in the same direction as the displacement. If this is not the case, then the work may be calculated as $W = Fd\cos(\theta)$, where θ is the angle between the force and displacement vectors. If force and displacement have the same direction, then work is positive; if they are in opposite directions, then work is negative; and if they are perpendicular, the work done by the force is zero.

As an example, if a man pushes a block horizontally across a surface with a constant force of 10 N for a distance of 20 m, the work done by the man is 200 N-m or 200 J. If instead the block is sliding and the man tries to slow its progress by pushing against it, his work done is -200 J, since he is pushing in the direction opposite the motion. If the man pushes vertically downward on the block while it slides, his work done is zero, since his force vector is perpendicular to the displacement vector of the block.

> ➤ **Review Video: Work**
> *Visit **mometrix.com/academy** and enter **Code: 681834***

Friction

Friction is a force that arises as a resistance to motion where two surfaces are in contact. The maximum magnitude of the frictional force (f)can be calculated as $f = F_c\mu$, where F_c is the contact force between the two objects and μ is a coefficient of friction based on the surfaces' material composition. Two types of friction are static and kinetic. To illustrate these concepts, imagine a book resting on a table. The force of its weight (W) is equal and opposite to the force of the table on the book, or the normal force (N). If we exert a small force (F) on the book, attempting to push it to one side, a frictional force (f) would arise, equal and opposite to our force. At this point, it is a *static frictional force* because the book is not moving. If we increase our force on the book, we will eventually cause it to move. At this point, the frictional force opposing us will be a *kinetic frictional force*. Generally, the kinetic frictional force is lower than static frictional force (because the frictional coefficient for static friction is larger), which means that the amount of force needed to maintain the movement of the book will be less than what was needed to start it moving.

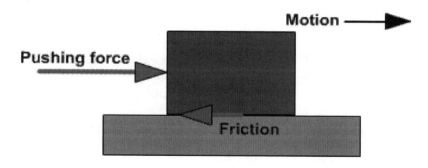

> ➤ **Review Video: Friction**
> *Visit **mometrix.com/academy** and enter **Code: 716782***

Gravitational force

Gravitational force is a universal force that causes every object to exert a force on every other object. The gravitational force between two objects can be described by the formula, $F = Gm_1m_2/r^2$, where m_1 and m_2 are the masses of two objects, r is the distance between them, and G is the gravitational constant, $G = 6.672 \times 10^{-11}$ N-m^2/kg^2.

In order for this force to have a noticeable effect, one or both of the objects must be extremely large, so the equation is generally only used in problems involving planetary bodies. For problems involving objects on the earth being affected by earth's gravitational pull, the force of gravity is simply calculated as F = mg, where g is 9.81 m/s^2 toward the ground.

Electrical force

Electrical force is a universal force that exists between any two electrically charged objects. Opposite charges attract one another and like charges repel one another. The magnitude of the force is directly proportional to the magnitude of the charges (q)and inversely proportional to the square of the distance (r) between the two objects: $F = kq_1q_2/r^2$, where $k = 9 \times 10^9$ N-m^2/C^2. Magnetic forces operate on a similar principle.

Buoyancy

Archimedes's principle states that a buoyant (upward) force on a submerged object is equal to the weight of the liquid displaced by the object. Water has a density of one gram per cubic centimeter. Anything that floats in water has a lower density, and anything that sinks has a higher density. This principle of buoyancy can also be used to calculate the volume of an irregularly shaped object. The mass of the object (m) minus its apparent mass in the water (m_a) divided by the density of water (ρ_w), gives the object's volume: $V = (m-m_a)/\rho_w$.

Machines

Simple machines include the inclined plane, lever, wheel and axle, and pulley. These simple machines have no internal source of energy. More complex or compound machines can be formed from them. Simple machines provide a force known as a mechanical advantage and make it easier to accomplish a task. The inclined plane enables a force less than the object's weight to be used to push an object to a greater height. A lever enables a multiplication of force. The wheel and axle allows for movement with less resistance. Single or double pulleys allows for easier direction of force. The wedge and screw are forms of the inclined plane. A wedge turns a smaller force working over a greater distance into a larger force. The screw is similar to an incline that is wrapped around a shaft.

A certain amount of work is required to move an object. The amount cannot be reduced, but by changing the way the work is performed a mechanical advantage can be gained. A certain amount of work is required to raise an object to a given vertical height. By getting to a given height at an angle, the effort required is reduced, but the distance that must be traveled to reach a given height is increased.

An example of this is walking up a hill. One may take a direct, shorter, but steeper route, or one may take a more meandering, longer route that requires less effort. Examples of wedges include doorstops, axes, plows, zippers, and can openers.

A lever consists of a bar or plank and a pivot point or fulcrum. Work is performed by the bar, which swings at the pivot point to redirect the force. There are three types of levers: first, second, and third class. Examples of a first-class lever include balances, see-saws, nail extractors, and scissors (which also use wedges). In a second-class lever the fulcrum is placed at one end of the bar and the work is performed at the other end. The weight or load to be moved is in between. The closer to the fulcrum the weight is, the easier it is to move. Force is increased, but the distance it is moved is decreased. Examples include pry bars, bottle openers, nutcrackers, and wheelbarrows. In a third-class lever the fulcrum is at one end and the positions of the weight and the location where the work is performed are reversed. Examples include fishing rods, hammers, and tweezers.

The center of a wheel and axle can be likened to a fulcrum on a rotating lever. As it turns, the wheel moves a greater distance than the axle, but with less force. Obvious examples of the wheel and axle are the wheels of a car, but this type of simple machine can also be used to exert a greater force. For instance, a person can turn the handles of a winch to exert a greater force at the turning axle to move an object. Other examples include steering wheels, wrenches, faucets, waterwheels, windmills, gears, and belts. Gears work together to change a force. The four basic types of gears are spur, rack and pinion, bevel, and worm gears. The larger gear turns slower than the smaller, but exerts a greater force. Gears at angles can be used to change the direction of forces.

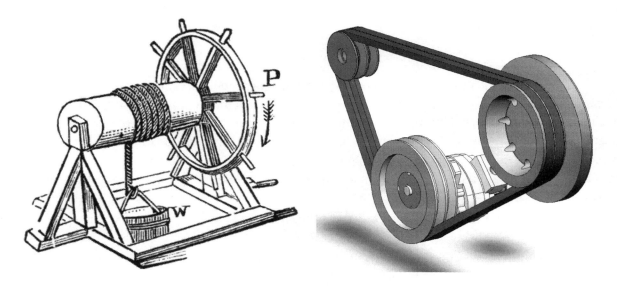

A single pulley consists of a rope or line that is run around a wheel. This allows force to be directed in a downward motion to lift an object. This does not decrease the force required, just changes its direction. The load is moved the same distance as the rope pulling it. When a combination pulley is used, such as a double pulley, the weight is moved half the distance of the rope pulling it. In this way, the work effort is doubled. Pulleys are never 100% efficient because of friction. Examples of pulleys include cranes, chain hoists, block and tackles, and elevators.

Electrical Charges

A glass rod and a plastic rod can illustrate the concept of static electricity due to friction. Both start with no charge. A glass rod rubbed with silk produces a positive charge, while a plastic rod rubbed with fur produces a negative charge. The electron affinity of a material is a property that helps determine how easily it can be charged by friction. Materials can be sorted by their affinity for electrons into a triboelectric series. Materials with greater affinities include celluloid, sulfur, and rubber. Materials with lower affinities include glass, rabbit fur, and asbestos. In the example of a glass rod and a plastic one, the glass rod rubbed with silk acquires a positive charge because glass has a lower affinity for electrons than silk. The electrons flow to the silk, leaving the rod with fewer electrons and a positive charge. When a plastic rod is rubbed with fur, electrons flow to the rod and result in a negative charge.

The attractive force between the electrons and the nucleus is called the electric force. A positive (+) charge or a negative (-) charge creates a field of sorts in the empty space around it, which is known as an electric field. The direction of a positive charge is away from it and the direction of a negative charge is towards it. An electron within the force of the field is pulled towards a positive charge because an electron has a negative charge. A particle with a positive charge is pushed away, or repelled, by another positive charge. Like charges repel each other and opposite charges attract. Lines of force show the paths of charges. Electric force between two objects is directly proportional to the product of the charge magnitudes and inversely proportional to the square of the distance between the two objects. Electric charge is measured with the unit Coulomb (C). It is the amount of charge moved in one second by a steady current of one ampere (1C = 1A × 1s).

Insulators are materials that prevent the movement of electrical charges, while conductors are materials that allow the movement of electrical charges. This is because conductive materials have free electrons that can move through the entire volume of the conductor. This allows an external charge to change the charge distribution in the material. In induction, a neutral conductive material, such as a sphere, can become charged by a positively or negatively charged object, such as a rod. The charged object is placed close to the material without touching it. This produces a force on the free electrons, which will either be attracted to or repelled by the rod, polarizing (or separating) the charge. The sphere's electrons will flow into or out of it when touched by a ground. The sphere is now charged. The charge will be opposite that of the charging rod.

Charging by conduction is similar to charging by induction, except that the material transferring the charge actually touches the material receiving the charge. A negatively or positively charged object is touched to an object with a neutral charge. Electrons will either flow into or out of the neutral object and it will become charged. Insulators cannot be used to conduct charges. Charging by conduction can also be called charging by contact.

The law of conservation of charge states that the total number of units before and after a charging process remains the same. No electrons have been created. They have just been moved around. The removal of a charge on an object by conduction is called grounding.

Circuits

Electric potential, or electrostatic potential or voltage, is an expression of potential energy per unit of charge. It is measured in volts (V) as a scalar quantity. The formula used is $V = E/Q$, where V is voltage, E is electrical potential energy, and Q is the charge. Voltage is typically discussed in the context of electric potential difference between two points in a circuit. Voltage can also be thought of as a measure of the rate at which energy is drawn from a source in order to produce a flow of electric charge.

Electric current is the sustained flow of electrons that are part of an electric charge moving along a path in a circuit. This differs from a static electric charge, which is a constant non-moving charge rather than a continuous flow. The rate of flow of electric charge is expressed using the ampere (amp or A) and can be measured using an ammeter. A current of 1 ampere means that 1 coulomb of charge passes through a given area every second. Electric charges typically only move from areas of high electric potential to areas of low electric potential. To get charges to flow into a high potential area, you must to connect it to an area of higher potential, by introducing a battery or other voltage source.

Electric currents experience resistance as they travel through a circuit. Different objects have different levels of resistance. The ohm (Ω) is the measurement unit of electric resistance. The symbol is the Greek letter omega. Ohm's Law, which is expressed as $I = V/R$, states that current flow (I, measured in amps) through an object is equal to the potential difference from one side to the other (V, measured in volts) divided by resistance (R, measured in ohms). An object with a higher resistance will have a lower current flow through it given the same potential difference.

Movement of electric charge along a path between areas of high electric potential and low electric potential, with a resistor or load device between them, is the definition of a simple circuit. It is a closed conducting path between the high and low potential points, such as the positive and negative terminals on a battery. One example of a circuit is the flow from one terminal of a car battery to the other. The electrolyte solution of water and sulfuric acid provides work in chemical form to start the flow. A frequently used classroom example of circuits involves using a D cell (1.5 V) battery, a small light bulb, and a piece of copper wire to create a circuit to light the bulb.

> **Review Video: Circuits**
*Visit **mometrix.com/academy** and enter Code: **472696***

Magnets

A magnet is a piece of metal, such as iron, steel, or magnetite (lodestone) that can affect another substance within its field of force that has like characteristics. Magnets can either attract or repel other substances. Magnets have two poles: north and south. Like poles repel and opposite poles (pairs of north and south) attract. The magnetic field is a set of invisible lines representing the paths of attraction and repulsion. Magnetism can occur naturally, or ferromagnetic materials can be magnetized. Certain matter that is magnetized can retain its magnetic properties indefinitely and become a permanent magnet. Other matter can lose its magnetic properties. For example, an iron nail can be temporarily magnetized by stroking it repeatedly in the same direction using one pole of another magnet. Once magnetized, it can attract or repel other magnetically inclined materials, such as paper clips. Dropping the nail repeatedly will cause it to lose its charge.

The motions of subatomic structures (nuclei and electrons) produce a magnetic field. It is the direction of the spin and orbit that indicate the direction of the field. The strength of a magnetic field is known as the magnetic moment. As electrons spin and orbit a nucleus, they produce a magnetic field. Pairs of electrons that spin and orbit in opposite directions cancel each other out, creating a net magnetic field of zero. Materials that have an unpaired electron are magnetic. Those with a weak attractive force are referred to as paramagnetic materials, while ferromagnetic materials have a strong attractive force. A diamagnetic material has electrons that are paired, and therefore does not typically have a magnetic moment. There are, however, some diamagnetic materials that have a weak magnetic field.

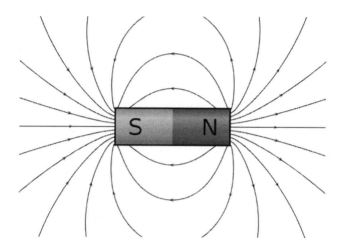

A magnetic field can be formed not only by a magnetic material, but also by electric current flowing through a wire. When a coiled wire is attached to the two ends of a battery, for example, an electromagnet can be formed by inserting a ferromagnetic material such as an iron bar within the coil. When electric current flows through the wire, the bar becomes a magnet. If there is no current, the magnetism is lost. A magnetic domain occurs when the magnetic fields of atoms are grouped and aligned. These groups form what can be thought of as miniature magnets within a material. This is what happens when an object like an iron nail is temporarily magnetized. Prior to magnetization, the organization of atoms and their various polarities are somewhat random with respect to where the north and south poles are pointing. After magnetization, a significant percentage of the poles are lined up in one direction, which is what causes the magnetic force exerted by the material.

➤ **Review Video: <u>Magnets</u>**
*Visit **mometrix.com/academy** and enter **Code: 570803***

Waves

Waves have energy and can transfer energy when they interact with matter. Although waves transfer energy, they do not transport matter. They are a disturbance of matter that transfers energy from one particle to an adjacent particle. There are many types of waves, including sound, seismic, water, light, micro, and radio waves. The two basic categories of waves are mechanical and electromagnetic. Mechanical waves are those that transmit energy through matter. Electromagnetic waves can transmit energy through a vacuum. A transverse wave provides a good illustration of the features of a wave, which include crests, troughs, amplitude, and wavelength. There are a number of important attributes of waves.

Frequency is a measure of how often particles in a medium vibrate when a wave passes through the medium with respect to a certain point or node. Usually measured in Hertz (Hz), frequency might refer to cycles per second, vibrations per second, or waves per second. One Hz is equal to one cycle per second.

Period is a measure of how long it takes to complete a cycle. It is the inverse of frequency; where frequency is measure in cycles per second, period can be thought of as seconds per cycle, though it is measured in units of time only.

Speed refers to how fast or slow a wave travels. It is measured in terms of distance divided by time. While frequency is measured in terms of cycles per second, speed might be measured in terms of meters per second.

Amplitude is the maximum amount of displacement of a particle in a medium from its rest position, and corresponds to the amount of energy carried by the wave. High energy waves have greater amplitudes; low energy waves have lesser amplitudes. Amplitude is a measure of a wave's strength.

Rest position, also called equilibrium, is the point at which there is neither positive nor negative displacement. Crest, also called the peak, is the point at which a wave's positive or upward displacement from the rest position is at its maximum. Trough, also called a valley, is the point at which a wave's negative or downward displacement from the rest position is at its maximum. A wavelength is one complete wave cycle. It could be measured from crest to crest, trough to trough, rest position to rest position, or any point of a wave to the corresponding point on the next wave.

Sound is a pressure disturbance that moves through a medium in the form of mechanical waves, which transfer energy from one particle to the next. Sound requires a medium to travel through, such as air, water, or other matter since it is the vibrations that transfer energy to adjacent particles, not the actual movement of particles over a great distance. Sound is transferred through the movement of atomic particles, which can be atoms or molecules. Waves of sound energy move outward in all directions from the source. Sound waves consist of compressions (particles are forced together) and rarefactions (particles move farther apart and their density decreases). A wavelength consists of one compression and one rarefaction. Different sounds have different wavelengths. Sound is a form of kinetic energy.

The electromagnetic spectrum is defined by frequency (f) and wavelength (λ). Frequency is typically measured in hertz and wavelength is usually measured in meters. Because light travels at a fairly constant speed, frequency is inversely proportional to wavelength, a relationship expressed by the formula $f = c/\lambda$, where c is the speed of light (about 300 million meters per second).

Frequency multiplied by wavelength equals the speed of the wave; for electromagnetic waves, this is the speed of light, with some variance for the medium in which it is traveling. Electromagnetic waves include (from largest to smallest wavelength) radio waves, microwaves, infrared radiation (radiant heat), visible light, ultraviolet radiation, x-rays, and gamma rays. The energy of electromagnetic waves is carried in packets that have a magnitude inversely proportional to the wavelength. Radio waves have a range of wavelengths, from about 10^{-3} to 10^5 meters, while their frequencies range from 10^3 to about 10^{11} Hz.

Atoms and molecules can gain or lose energy only in particular, discrete amounts. Therefore, they can absorb and emit light only at wavelengths that correspond to these amounts. Using a process known as spectroscopy, these characteristic wavelengths can be used to identify substances.

Light is the portion of the electromagnetic spectrum that is visible because of its ability to stimulate the retina. It is absorbed and emitted by electrons, atoms, and molecules that move from one energy level to another. Visible light interacts with matter through molecular electron excitation (which occurs in the human retina) and through plasma oscillations (which occur in metals). Visible light is between ultraviolet and infrared light on the spectrum. The wavelengths of visible light cover a range from 380 nm (violet) to 760 nm (red). Different wavelengths correspond to different colors. The human brain interprets or perceives visible light, which is emitted from the sun and other stars, as color. For example, when the entire wavelength reaches the retina, the brain perceives the color white. When no part of the wavelength reaches the retina, the brain perceives the color black.

When light waves encounter an object, they are either reflected, transmitted, or absorbed. If the light is reflected from the surface of the object, the angle at which it contacts the surface will be the same as the angle at which it leaves, on the other side of the perpendicular. If the ray of light is perpendicular to the surface, it will be reflected back in the direction from which it came. When light is transmitted through the object, its direction may be altered upon entering the object. This is known as refraction. The degree to which the light is refracted depends on the speed at which light travels in the object. Light that is neither reflected nor transmitted will be absorbed by the surface and stored as heat energy. Nearly all instances of light hitting an object will involve a combination of two or even all three of these.

When light waves are refracted, or bent, an image can appear distorted. Sound waves and water waves can also be refracted. Diffraction refers to the bending of waves around small objects and the spreading out of waves past small openings. The narrower the opening, the greater the level of diffraction will be. Larger wavelengths also increase diffraction. A diffraction grating can be created by placing a number of slits close together, and is used more frequently than a prism to separate light. Different wavelengths are diffracted at different angles. The particular color of an object depends upon what is absorbed and what is transmitted or reflected.

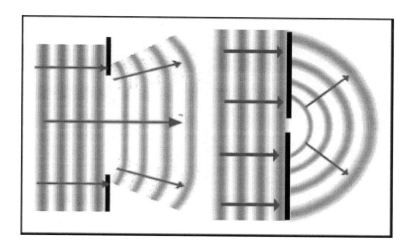

For example, a leaf consists of chlorophyll molecules, the atoms of which absorb all wavelengths of the visible light spectrum except for green, which is why a leaf appears green. Certain wavelengths of visible light can be absorbed when they interact with matter. Wavelengths that are not absorbed can be transmitted by transparent materials or reflected by opaque materials.

The various properties of light have numerous real life applications. For example, polarized sunglasses have lenses that help reduce glare, while non-polarized sunglasses reduce the total amount of light that reaches the eyes. Polarized lenses consist of a chemical film of molecules aligned in parallel. This allows the lenses to block wavelengths of light that are intense, horizontal, and reflected from smooth, flat surfaces. The "fiber" in fiber optics refers to a tube or pipe that channels light. Because of the composition of the fiber, light can be transmitted greater distances before losing the signal. The fiber consists of a core, cladding, and a coating. Fibers are bundled, allowing for the transmission of large amounts of data.

Part V. – Vocational Adjustment Index

This is a mini-test that evaluates your opinions and attitudes related to the nursing profession and practice as a professional. You cannot prepare for this section of the exam. You will be asked questions on quality of care, delivery of services, and patient rights. Moreover, the goal of this mini-test is to determine your opinions about professional care. If you answer with "extreme" points of view, you will not be scored well on this assessment.

Practice Test

Academic Aptitude

Verbal

In the following sets of words, choose the word that is most different in meaning from the others.

1. a. Expand   b. Contract   c. Shrink   d. Diminish   e. Lessen

2. a. Abhor   b. Adore   c. Despise   d. Hate   e. Deplore

3. a. Trite   b. Cliché   c. Original   d. Overused   e. Commonplace

4. a. Bicker   b. Argue   c. Quarrel   d. Cooperate   e. Disagree

5. a. Pandemonium   b. Chaos   c. Excitement   d. Disarray   e. Harmony

6. a. Somber   b. Gleeful   c. Serious   d. Sad   e. Gloomy

7. a. Apprehension   b. Trepidation   c. Optimism   d. Dread   e. Anxiety

8. a. Dismal   b. Dreary   c. Bleak   d. Cheery   e. Depressing

9. a. Fortunate   b. Hapless   c. Unlucky   d. Tragic   e. Doomed

10. a. Disperse   b. Thin   c. Collect   d. Dissipate   e. Scatter

11. a. Oblivious   b. Clueless   c. Aware   d. Heedless   e. Ignorant

12. a. Distraught   b. Alarmed   c. Agitated   d. Tranquil   e. Distracted

13. a. Bedlam   b. Confusion   c. Havoc   d. Uproar   e. Order

14. a. Ambiguous   b. Clear   c. Vague   d. Arcane   e. Cryptic

15. a. Invite   b. Avert   c. Evade   d. Prevent   e. Elude

16. a. Unique   b. Mundane   c. Ordinary   d. Quotidian   e. Pedestrian

17. a. Perpetual   b. Constant   c. Occasional   d. Ceaseless   e. Running

18. a. Vexing   b. Gratifying   c. Irritating   d. Annoying   e. Aggravating

19. a. Sagacious   b. Wise   c. Knowing   d. Ignorant   e. Astute

20. a. Audacious   b. Bold   c. Brash   d. Rude   e. Humble

21. a. Deriding   b. Approving   c. Praising   d. Favoring   e. Commending

22. a. Stealthy   b. Secretive   c. Sneaky   d. Sly   e. Transparent

23. a. Impudent   b. Impertinent   c. Respectful   d. Rude   e. Sassy

24. a. Blissful   b. Blithe   c. Jubilant   d. Aggrieved   e. Jocund

25. a. Gaunt   b. Plump   c. Haggard   d. Wasted   e. Skinny

26. a. Unassuming   b. Haughty   c. Superior   d. Lofty   e. Presumptuous

27. a. Blasphemous   b. Reverent   c. Profane   d. Impious   e. Sacrilegious

28. a. Heretic   b. Renegade   c. Believer   d. Defector   e. Dissident

29. a. Cynical   b. Trusting   c. Skeptical   d. Suspicious   e. Pessimistic

30. a. Agape   b. Anticipating   c. Eager   d. Unmoved   e. Agog

Arithmetic

1. 236
 +301
    a. 505
    b. 507
    c. 535
    d. 537

2. 4,307
 +1,864
    a. 5,161
    b. 5,271
    c. 6,171
    d. 6,271

3. If $a = 3$ and $b = -2$, what is the value of $a^2 + 3ab - b^2$?
    a. 5
    b. -13
    c. -4
    d. -20

4. 356
 - 167
    a. 189
    b. 198
    c. 211
    d. 298

5. 5,306
 -3,487
    a. 1,181
    b. 1,819
    c. 2,119
    d. 2,189

6. 34 is what percent of 80?
    a. 34%
    b. 40%
    c. 42.5%
    d. 44.5%

7. 707
 x 17
    a. 12,019
    b. 12,049
    c. 17,019
    d. 17,049

8. $7\overline{)917}$
    a. 131
    b. 131 R4
    c. 145
    d. 145 R4

9. Factor the following expression: $x^2 + x - 12$
    a. $(x - 4)\ (x + 4)$
    b. $(x - 2)\ (x + 6)$
    c. $(x + 6)\ (x - 2)$
    d. $(x + 4)\ (x - 3)$

10. $\frac{38}{100}$ as a decimal
    a. 0.38
    b. 0.038
    c. 3.8
    d. 0.0038

11.
$$
\begin{array}{r}
6.8 \\
11.3 \\
+\ \ \ 0.06 \\
\hline
\end{array}
$$
    a. 17.16
    b. 17.70
    c. 18.16
    d. 18.70

12. The average of six numbers is 4. If the average of two of those numbers is 2, what is the average of the other four numbers?
    a. 5
    b. 6
    c. 7
    d. 8

13. Which numeral is in the thousandths place in 0.3874?
    a. 3
    b. 8
    c. 7
    d. 4

14. 0.58 - 0.39=
    a. 0.19
    b. 1.9
    c. 0.29
    d. 2.9

15. Solve: 0.25 x 0.03 =
   a. 75
   b. 0.075
   c. 0.75
   d. 0.0075

16. $3\frac{1}{8} + 6 + \frac{3}{7} =$

   a. $9\frac{31}{56}$

   b. $9\frac{1}{2}$

   c. $9\frac{21}{56}$

   d. $9\frac{7}{8}$

17. $4\frac{1}{7} - 2\frac{1}{2} =$

   a. $2\frac{5}{14}$

   b. $1\frac{5}{14}$

   c. $1\frac{9}{14}$

   d. $2\frac{9}{14}$

18. $1\frac{1}{4} \times 3\frac{2}{5} \times 1\frac{2}{3} =$

   a. $7\frac{1}{12}$

   b. $5\frac{5}{6}$

   c. $6\frac{7}{12}$

   d. $8\frac{11}{15}$

19. How many 3-inch segments can a 4.5-yard line be divided into?
   a. 15
   b. 45
   c. 54
   d. 64

20. Reduce $\frac{14}{98}$ to lowest terms.

   a. $\frac{7}{49}$

   b. $\frac{2}{14}$

   c. $\frac{1}{7}$

   d. $\frac{3}{8}$

21. Thirty six hundredths as a percent.
    a. 36%
    b. 0.36%
    c. 0.036%
    d. 3.6%

22. 40% of 900
    a. 280
    b. 340
    c. 360
    d. 420

23. Sheila, Janice, and Karen, working together at the same rate, can complete a job in 3 1/3 days. Working at the same rate, how much of the job could Janice and Karen do in one day?
    a. $\frac{1}{5}$
    b. $\frac{1}{4}$
    c. $\frac{1}{3}$
    d. $\frac{1}{9}$

24. Three eighths of forty equals:
    a. 15
    b. 20
    c. 22
    d. 24

25. 6% of 25
    a. .3
    b. 1.5
    c. 3.0
    d. 15

26. Ratio of 4 to 16 = (?)%
    a. 2
    b. 4
    c. 12
    d. 25

27. $4^6 \div 2^8 =$
    a. 2
    b. 8
    c. 16
    d. 32

28. 30% as a reduced common fraction

    a. $\frac{30}{100}$

    b. $\frac{1}{30}$

    c. $\frac{23}{10}$

    d. $\frac{3}{10}$

29. 37% as a decimal
    a. .0037
    b. .037
    c. .37
    d. 3.7

30. $-4a + 6a + 2a$
    a. $4a$
    b. $-4a$
    c. $8a$
    d. $12a$

Nonverbal

For each question, there is a relationship between the first two figures presented, and then a third figure is presented. Find the answer choice that relates to the third figure in the same way that the first two figures are related.

1. [symbol] is to [symbol] as [symbol] is to?   a. [symbol]   b. [symbol]   c. [symbol]   d. [symbol]   e. [symbol]

2. [symbol] is to [symbol] as [symbol] is to?   a. [symbol]   b. [symbol]   c. [symbol]   d. [symbol]   e. [symbol]

3. [symbol] is to [symbol] as [symbol] is to?   a. [symbol]   b. [symbol]   c. [symbol]   d. [symbol]   e. [symbol]

4. [symbol] is to [symbol] as [symbol] is to?   a. [symbol]   b. [symbol]   c. [symbol]   d. [symbol]   e. [symbol]

5. [symbol] is to [symbol] as [symbol] is to?   a. [symbol]   b. [symbol]   c. [symbol]   d. [symbol]   e. [symbol]

6. [symbol] is to [symbol] as [symbol] is to?   a. [symbol]   b. [symbol]   c. [symbol]   d. [symbol]   e. [symbol]

7. [symbol] is to [symbol] as [symbol] is to?   a. [symbol]   b. [symbol]   c. [symbol]   d. [symbol]   e. [symbol]

8. [symbol] is to [symbol] as [symbol] is to?   a. [symbol]   b. [symbol]   c. [symbol]   d. [symbol]   e. [symbol]

9. [symbol] is to [symbol] as [symbol] is to?   a. [symbol]   b. [symbol]   c. [symbol]   d. [symbol]   e. [symbol]

10. [symbol] is to [symbol] as [symbol] is to?   a. [symbol]   b. [symbol]   c. [symbol]   d. [symbol]   e. [symbol]

11. [symbol] is to [symbol] as [symbol] is to?   a. [symbol]   b. [symbol]   c. [symbol]   d. [symbol]   e. [symbol]

12. [symbol] is to [symbol] as [symbol] is to?   a. [symbol]   b. [symbol]   c. [symbol]   d. [symbol]   e. [symbol]

13. [symbol] is to [symbol] as [symbol] is to?   a. [symbol]   b. [symbol]   c. [symbol]   d. [symbol]   e. [symbol]

14. [symbol] to [symbol] as [symbol] is to?   a. [symbol]   b. [symbol]   c. [symbol]   d. [symbol]   e. [symbol]

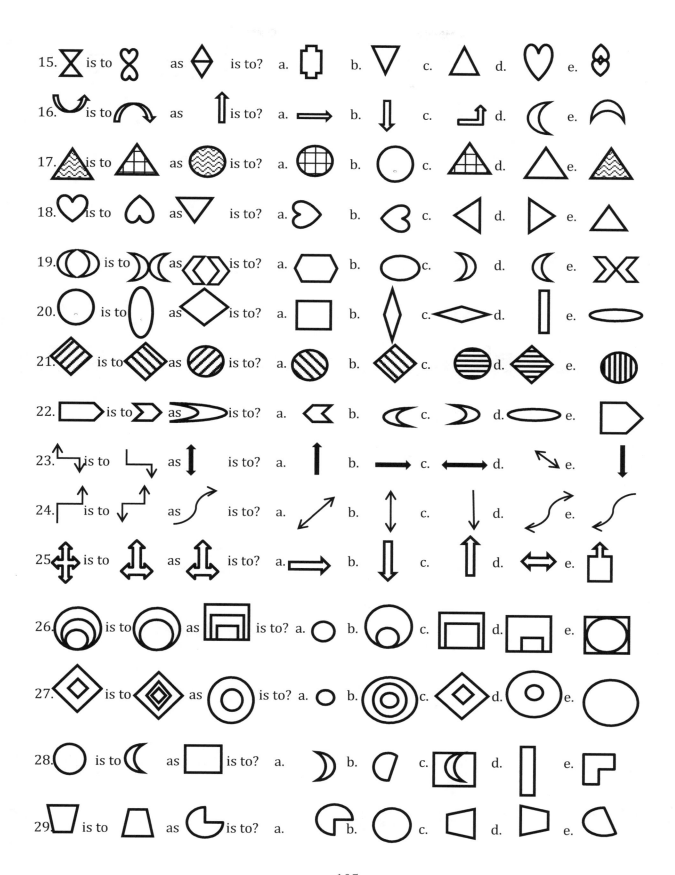

30. ⬭ is to ⬡ as △ is to?   a. ◇   b. ▽   c. ⬭   d. ⬡   e. ▽

Spelling

Each question gives three different spellings of a word. Two are incorrect and one is correct. Select the choice from each set of three that is spelled correctly.

1. a. separate   b. seperate   c. sepparate
2. a. nucular   b. nuclear   c. nuculear
3. a. fermiliar   b. farmiliar   c. familiar
4. a. sacrilegious   b. sacreligious   c. sacraligious
5. a. aggitated   b. agittated   c. agitated
6. a. orientated   b. oriented   c. oreinted
7. a. indispensible   b. indespensible   c. indispensable
8. a. similar   b. simular   c. similiar
9. a. atitude   b. attitude   c. atittude
10. a. abreviate   b. abbreviate   c. abreeviate
11. a. absorb   b. apsorb   c. abzorb
12. a. acumulate   b. acummulate   c. accumulate
13. a. airial   b. aireal   c. aerial
14. a. comedian   b. commedian   c. comedien
15. a. ashphalt   b. asphalt   c. aspalt
16. a. forceable   b. forcible   c. forceble
17. a. anicdote   b. antecdote   c. anecdote
18. a. flexible   b. flexable   c. flexiable
19. a. defendant   b. defendent   c. difendent
20. a. plainteff   b. plaintif   c. plaintiff
21. a. idiocincrasy   b. idiosyncrasy   c. idiosincracy
22. a. hazardous   b. hazerdous   c. hazzardous
23. a. horific   b. horrific   c. horriffic
24. a. hansome   b. handsom   c. handsome
25. a. liaison   b. liason   c. leiaison
26. a. galexy   b. galaxy   c. gallaxy
27. a. attorneys   b. atorneys   c. attornys
28. a. asteriks   b. asterix   c. asterisk
29. a. equalibrium   b. equilibrum   c. equilibrium
30. a. brilliance   b. brillance   c. briliance
31. a. blanche   b. blanch   c. blance
32. a. ecstasy   b. extasy   c. ecstacy
33. a. deppreciate   b. depreciate   c. deappreciate
34. a. terpitude   b. turpittude   c. turpitude
35. a. oposite   b. opposite   c. opossite
36. a. tyrrany   b. tyrranny   c. tyranny
37. a. schism   b. scism   c. shism
38. a. scedule   b. shedule   c. schedule
39. a. incandescent   b. incandesent   c. incandecent

40. a. teriffic	b. terrific	c. terriffic
41. a. homogeneize	b. homogenize	c. homoginise
42. a. sieve	b. seive	c. sive
43. a. truely	b. truley	c. truly
44. a. sincerely	b. sincerly	c. sinceerly
45. a. transeint	b. transient	c. transhent
46. a. sedition	b. sidition	c. sadition
47. a. theives	b. thiefs	c. thieves
48. a. vengance	b. vengeance	c. vengence
49. a. nilon	b. nylon	c. nyllon
50. a. unnacceptable	b. unaceptible	c. unacceptable
51. a. deficit	b. defecit	c. defficit
52. a. disaproval	b. disapproval	c. dissaproval
53. a. diffidence	b. difidence	c. diffedince
54. a. picknicking	b. picnicing	c. picnicking
55. a. oreggano	b. oreganno	c. oregano
56. a. batchelor	b. bachelor	c. bachler
57. a. indelible	b. indelable	c. indellible
58. a. dyurnal	b. diurnal	c. dayernal
59. a. impatience	b. impatiense	c. empatiance
60. a. parlament	b. parliment	c. parliament

Reading Comprehension

Read the following passage carefully. Answer questions 1–10 following the passage based on the information in the passage by choosing the correct answer from the four choices given. Work quickly but carefully.

It was moving day for the Robertson family. Bernard and Marian had married before World War II. Bernard was in the Army. When he returned from his tour of duty, the couple lived with Marian's widowed mother in the house her late husband had left to her. After several years they had a son, Lewis. Two years later they had a daughter, Hannah. When the children were seven and five years old respectively, their parents had both worked and saved up enough money to have a new house built. Now they were finally moving in, bringing along Marian's mother, whom the children called Nana, and their pet cat, whom they had named Fluffy.

The house was not completely finished, but it was livable. It was a hot summer day. After hours of setting up their furniture brought by the movers, and bringing in and unpacking many belongings, the family sat down to take a breather. Suddenly they noticed that Fluffy was missing. Fearing he had run outside during all the moving commotion and become lost in a new neighborhood, Marian and Hannah went walking around the block, calling their pet's name. Marian had contracted a terrible case of poison oak on her legs from petting Katie, a neighbor's beautiful Irish setter who had picked up the poison oak oils on her coat from running through the woods and then rubbed against Marian's bare legs. This made it painful for her to walk in the summer heat, but she was so worried about Fluffy. Hannah was equally distressed about her beloved pet.

After searching to no avail, the family decided to sit down to eat dinner and hope that Fluffy would show up at some point. Right in the middle of the meal, they heard a "Meow!" coming from the adjacent living room. Turning to look in the direction of the sound, they spotted Fluffy sitting on the hearth of their new fireplace! Excited, they all jumped up, shouting, "Fluffy!" Upon hearing the clamor, the little tabby immediately turned and jumped up into the chimney to escape. Now they realized that he had not been lost or outdoors at all, but had simply found a dark, quiet, cool place to hide from the commotion. Reaching up into the chimney, Bernard and Lewis discovered a ledge where Fluffy was comfortably perched. Marian offered up a little dish of hamburger, a favorite treat; but Fluffy just ate the meat without emerging from his hiding place. The family all laughed together at the kitty's cleverness and Mom's foolishness in not placing the meat farther away to lure him out of hiding.

The family agreed that it would be best to give their pet the safety and seclusion he needed after all the trauma of moving (cats generally hate any changes in their environment), and the noise and confusion of things being brought in and moved about, people coming in and going out, and so forth. They let him stay in the chimney. Once things had settled down and it was quiet in the house, Fluffy eventually came out of his safe refuge and began to explore his new surroundings. Soon he had adjusted to the new home. He slept on Hannah's bed, lounged on the living room chairs, kept Nana company while she sewed when the parents were at work and the children were at school, and scampered around the house playing. He had completely gotten over his initial fear and made himself at home with his family.

1. This story takes place:
   a. Several years after World War I.
   b. Several years after World War II.
   c. Several years after the Korean War.
   d. This information is not given in the story.

2. Nana was:
   a. What the children called their mother.
   b. The name the family gave to their cat.
   c. What the kids called their grandmother.
   d. The nickname the family called Hannah.

3. Marian contracted poison oak from:
   a. Running through the neighborhood woods.
   b. Petting their cat Fluffy who had it on his coat.
   c. Walking around the block in the summer heat.
   d. Having the dog Katie rub against her bare legs.

4. Before building their first new home, the Robertson family lived:
   a. In Nana's house.
   b. In an apartment.
   c. In another town.
   d. This is not given.

5. The "tour of duty" referred to in the passage means:
   a. The term that a soldier serves in the armed forces.
   b. A program of visiting various countries in the world.
   c. Fulfilling all the duties of moving into a new house.
   d. There is no such reference existing in this passage.

6. How did the family discover where Fluffy had been?
   a. He came to the dinner table, lured by the smell of meat.
   b. During dinner, they heard him meow from the living room.
   c. After hearing him, they saw him go back up the chimney.
   d. They walked around the block calling until they found him.

7. Why was Fluffy sitting on a ledge inside the chimney?
   a. Cats just naturally always hide.
   b. It was cooler on a summer day.
   c. To escape all the commotion.
   d. Both (B) and (C) are correct.

8. Which is the *least likely* reason Fluffy found moving day traumatic?
   a. Cats hate any changes in their environment.
   b. The moving process is noisy and confusing.
   c. There was a dog in the new neighborhood.
   d. It kept him from feeling privacy and safety.

9. Which of the following is NOT included among Fluffy's activities once he adjusted?
   a. Lounging on living room chairs
   b. Keeping Nana company sewing
   c. Climbing drapes in Lewis's room
   d. Sleeping in Hannah's bedroom

10. The <u>main</u> focus of this passage is:
    a. How the family lived with the grandmother in both homes.
    b. How hard two parents worked and saved to build a house.
    c. How difficult it was to move the family into the new home.
    d. How a family "lost" and then found their cat when moving.

Read the following passage carefully. Answer questions 11–20 following the passage based on the information in the passage by choosing the correct answer from the four choices given. Work quickly but carefully.

The phrase "boulevard of broken dreams" may be familiar to many people, because it has been used so often. In 1933, the songwriting team of lyricist Al Dubin and composer Harry Warren wrote a song entitled "Boulevard of Broken Dreams," which was a big hit in its day and, a version sung by Constance Bennett was included in the 1934 movie *Moulin Rouge.* The lyrics include the verses, "I walk along the street of sorrow/The Boulevard of Broken Dreams/Where gigolo and gigolette/Can take a kiss without regret/So they forget their broken dreams....Here is where you'll always find me/Always walking up and down...." Many other singers have covered this song over the years, including a 2006 duet by Tony Bennett and Sting, and some as recently as 2010 and 2012. The phrase "boulevard of broken dreams" was a reference to Sunset Boulevard in Los Angeles.

In 1942, the modern American artist Edward Hopper created an oil painting he called *Nighthawks.* It depicts a late-night scene of a diner in a downtown area. The street outside is deserted, and inside the lighted diner are three customers sitting at the counter and a man with a white hat and shirt behind the counter. This painting became very famous. What does this painting have to do with the phrase "boulevard of broken dreams"? Well, contemporary Viennese artist Gottfried Helnwein (born in 1948) created a parody of Hopper's painting in 1984. Helnwein's watercolor appears quite similar to Hopper's work—until you look more closely. Then you see that the anonymous people sitting in the diner in Hopper's original have been replaced in Helnwein's version with the iconic late celebrity actors Humphrey Bogart, Marilyn Monroe, and James Dean; and the attendant behind the counter has been replaced with the late Elvis Presley. These famous figures had all died young between 1955 and 1977.

Helnwein's was one of a number of parodies based on Hopper's painting. It inspired Billie Joe Armstrong, the lyricist and lead singer of the contemporary rock band Green Day, to write a song entitled "Boulevard of Broken Dreams." Its music and lyrics are different from the 1933 song: "I walk a lonely road/The only one that I have ever known/Don't know where it goes/But it's home to me and I walk alone/I walk alone, I walk alone...I walk this empty street/On the Boulevard of Broken Dreams/When the city sleeps/And I'm the only one and I walk alone/My shadow's

- 111 -

the only one that walks beside me/My shallow heart's the only thing that's beating/Sometimes I wish someone up there will find me/'til then I walk alone." Released in 2004 on their album *American Idiot*, the song became one of Green Day's biggest and most recognized hits.

Green Day was not the only example of works using the title "Boulevard of Broken Dreams." Country singer Ferlin Husky released an album with that title in 1957. The band Smokie released both an album and its title song with the same name in 1989. Songs with this title were also recorded by Juan García Esquivel (1958), Hanoi Rocks (1984), Brian Setzer (1986), David Cassidy (1990), Beatmasters (1991), and with the same title in Spanish by Joaquín Sabina (1994). In addition to painters and musicians, other artists have used the familiar phrase. Science fiction author Harlan Ellison entitled a 1978 short story "Boulevard of Broken Dreams," which he published in *Strange Wine*, a collection of his stories. An Australian movie with this title was released in 1988. Paul Alexander published a biography of James Dean entitled *Boulevard of Broken Dreams* (1994)—perhaps inspired by Dean's likeness in Helnwein's painting. Kim Deitch published an acclaimed graphic novel (2002) with the same title. In 2007, the E! television network aired a documentary series about celebrities, also using this title.

11. The earliest use of the title and lyric "Boulevard of Broken Dreams" identified in the passage was by:
    a. Billie Joe Armstrong
    b. Tony Bennett and Sting
    c. Al Dubin and Harry Warren
    d. Gottfried Helnwein

12. The famous painting by Edward Hopper described in the passage is entitled:
    a. *Boulevard of Broken Dreams*
    b. *American Idiot*
    c. *Strange Wine*
    d. *Nighthawks*

13. In the movie *Moulin Rouge,* a song entitled "Boulevard of Broken Dreams" is sung by:
    a. Constance Bennett
    b. Tony Bennett and Sting
    c. Billie Joe and Green Day
    d. Juan García Esquivel

14. Which is correct about the media used by two painters described in the passage?
    a. Hopper used watercolors, and Helnwein used oils.
    b. Hopper used oils, and Helnwein used watercolors.
    c. Both Hopper and Helnwein used oils in their work.
    d. Both Hopper and Helnwein used watercolor paint.

15. According to the passage, who wrote the lyrics "I walk alone, I walk alone"?
    a. Al Dubin
    b. Harry Warren
    c. Constance Bennett
    d. Billie Joe Armstrong

16. Which celebrities are portrayed in Edward Hopper's famous painting?
    a. James Dean
    b. Elvis Presley
    c. Marilyn Monroe
    d. None of these.

17. Related to "Boulevard of Broken Dreams," which of the following occurred earliest in time?
    a. Paul Alexander wrote a biography of James Dean with this title.
    b. Kim Deitch published an acclaimed graphic novel using this title.
    c. Harlan Ellison published a science fiction story that had the title.
    d. E! television network aired a documentary series with this title.

18. Green Day's hit song was inspired by:
    a. The famous painting by Edward Hopper.
    b. The Hopper parody by Gottfried Helnwein.
    c. The 1933 song by Al Dubin and Harry Warren.
    d. The movie *Moulin Rouge*, first released in 1934.

19. The title "Boulevard of Broken Dreams" has been used in:
    a. Paintings, songs, albums, movies, books, and TV.
    b. Many individual songs, but never in any albums.
    c. Movies and a TV series, but never in any books.
    d. Paintings and songs, but never in books or TV.

20. The celebrities depicted in the painting:
    a. Had all been dead for years when the painting was made.
    b. Had all just recently died when the painting was created.
    c. Were all still alive at the time the artist made the painting.
    d. Cannot be determined as dead or alive from this passage.

Read the following passage carefully. Answer questions 21–30 following the passage based on the information in the passage by choosing the correct answer from the four choices given. Work quickly but carefully.

Imidacloprid is a chemical pesticide, one of the most commonly used on the planet. It is the active ingredient in Advantage™, used to kill fleas on pets. It is chemically related to nicotine. It acts on the central nervous systems of insects by blocking neurons from taking up the brain chemical acetylcholine, which is necessary for their muscles to work. It has also been found to disrupt bees' internal navigating systems, and their communicative dance that informs their hive of food locations. Imidacloprid is used in homes to control termites, cockroaches, carpenter ants, and other pests, and in gardens to control aphids, beetles, and other insects. It is widely used in agriculture to protect trees and food crops from insect damage.

The biggest farm crop in America is corn. Imidacloprid has been used to treat most of our cornfields since 2004. In addition to feeding farm livestock and people, corn is also used to make high-fructose corn syrup. This syrup is ubiquitously found in an enormous number of commercial food products—not only sweetened soft drinks and desserts, but also breads, frozen meals, and many other foods. Research has found that the pesticide Imidacloprid moves from germinating corn seeds into the plants, and then into the kernels of the corn. Therefore, the majority of Americans are ingesting this chemical.

Beginning in 2006, farmers and scientists observed that honeybee populations were declining dramatically, on the order of about 30% per year. This decline was so striking that scientists have named it "bee colony collapse disorder." At first they did not know what was causing it; but it was considered a serious problem for agriculture, because the United States Department of Agriculture (USDA) estimates that more than $15 billion a year in crop values is attributed to the pollination of crop plants by honeybees.

Dr. Chensheng Lu, an environmental biologist working at Emory University in 2006, studied the exposure of children to pesticides in foods. He found metabolites of organophosphates, chemicals used in pesticides, in school children's urine. He additionally found that when their diets were changed to organic produce, grown without pesticide use, these substances disappeared from the children's urine right away.

In 2010, Lu, who had moved to the Harvard School of Public Health, conducted a study in environmental exposure biology. He suspected the pesticide imidacloprid might be implicated in the vanishing bee populations. During the winter, high-fructose corn syrup is commonly used to feed honeybees as a much cheaper substitute for honey. In the summer, Lu established beehives in four different locations. At each site, 1 of 5 hives, the control, was fed plain high-fructose corn syrup; the other four, experimental hives each received high-fructose corn syrup with various amounts of imidacloprid. The results were significant: within 13 weeks, two hives of bees were dead; and within 23 weeks, 15 out of 16 experimental (pesticide-treated) hives were dead. Other than one hive that died from a dysentery outbreak, none of the control hives given corn syrup without imidacloprid died. Although the hives getting the highest doses of imidacloprid died most quickly, another significant finding was that bees also died from doses lower than those they would get from their normal crop foraging.

Because high-fructose corn syrup is not directly marketed to consumers, levels of imidacloprid residues in it are not monitored as they are in foods. But most Americans consume a lot of this H-F corn syrup in other foods. Therefore, Dr. Lu has made the point that human health problems can be caused by low doses of pesticides in foods. However, he has added that no data to prove this have been gathered from studies of humans. He has stated that lacking plenty of such data from humans, imidacloprid can continue to be approved for use for 20 or 30 years longer.

21. According to the passage, for what purpose is imidacloprid NOT used?
   a. Killing fleas on pets
   b. Killing garden pests
   c. Protecting farm crops
   d. Nicotine substitute

22. Americans are ingesting imidacloprid through:
    a. Eating it in corn kernels.
    b. Inhaling it from the air.
    c. High-fructose corn syrup.
    d. Both answers A and C.

23. Dr. Chensheng Lu has been doing research in the 2000s at:
    a. Emory University.
    b. Harvard University.
    c. Both of these.
    d. Neither one.

24. Dr. Lu's research has found that the cause of bee colony collapse disorder:
    a. Still remains a complete mystery to this day.
    b. Includes factors too numerous to mention.
    c. Is associated with the use of imidacloprid.
    d. Comes from feeding bees H-F corn syrup.

25. The pesticide discussed kills insects by:
    a. Destroying their brain neurons.
    b. Disrupting acetylcholine uptake.
    c. Introducing toxic acetylcholine.
    d. The mechanism is not known.

26. In Lu's 2006 experiment, which of these happened?
    a. Chemicals persisted in children's urine despite organic diets.
    b. Organic diets made pesticide residues disappear right away.
    c. School children fed diets with high-fructose corn syrup died.
    d. Beehive populations fed on high-fructose corn syrup all died.

27. In Lu's 2010 experiment, which of these happened?
    a. Beehives fed imidacloprid-laced H-F corn syrup in summer died.
    b. Beehives fed high-fructose corn syrup during the winter all died.
    c. School children fed imidacloprid-laced H-F corn syrup became ill.
    d. Both beehives and school children were harmed by imidacloprid.

28. A significant conclusion Dr. Lu made from his research results was:
    a. Even low doses of pesticide can cause human health problems.
    b. Only very high doses of pesticides cause human health issues.
    c. Pesticide in corn syrup kills bees, but does not affect humans.
    d. The use of imidacloprid on crops must be banned immediately.

29. Which of the following is true about monitoring chemical levels in foods?
    a. There is no monitoring of the levels of any chemical residues in foods.
    b. Government agencies monitor levels of all chemical residues in foods.
    c. Chemical residues are monitored in foods, but not in H-F corn syrup.
    d. H-F corn syrup is monitored because it is sold directly to consumers.

30. Which of the following is a conclusion of Dr. Lu related in the passage?
    a. Imidacloprid use on crops will be discontinued very soon.
    b. Imidacloprid use may be approved for 20–30 more years.
    c. Imidacloprid use does not harm bees at very low levels.
    d. There is abundant data on imidacloprid effects on humans.

Natural Science

1. What is the name for any substance that stimulates the production of antibodies?
    a. collagen
    b. hemoglobin
    c. lymph
    d. antigen

2. Which of the following correctly lists the cellular hierarchy from the simplest to the most complex structure?
    a. tissue, cell, organ, organ system, organism
    b. organism, organ system, organ, tissue, cell
    c. organ system, organism, organ, tissue, cell
    d. cell, tissue, organ, organ system, organism

3. If a cell is placed in a hypertonic solution, what will happen to the cell?
    a. It will swell.
    b. It will shrink.
    c. It will stay the same.
    d. It does not affect the cell.

4. Which group of major parts and organs make up the immune system?
    a. lymphatic system, spleen, tonsils, thymus, and bone marrow
    b. brain, spinal cord, and nerve cells
    c. heart, veins, arteries, and capillaries
    d. nose, trachea, bronchial tubes, lungs, alveolus, and diaphragm

5. The rate of a chemical reaction depends on all of the following except
    a. temperature
    b. surface area.
    c. presence of catalysts.
    d. amount of mass lost.

6. Which of the answer choices provided best defines the following statement?
For a given mass and constant temperature, an inverse relationship exists between the volume and pressure of a gas.
    a. Ideal Gas Law
    b. Boyle's Law
    c. Charles' Law
    d. Stefan-Boltzmann Law

7. Which of the following statements correctly compares prokaryotic and eukaryotic cells?
    a. Prokaryotic cells have a true nucleus, eukaryotic cells do not.
    b. Both prokaryotic and eukaryotic cells have a membrane.
    c. Prokaryotic cells do not contain membrane-bound organelles, eukaryotic cells do.
    d. Prokaryotic cells are more complex than eukaryotic cells.

8. What is the role of ribosomes?
    a. make proteins
    b. waste removal
    c. transport
    d. storage

9. If an organism is *AaBb*, which of the following combinations in the gametes is impossible?
    a. AB
    b. aa
    c. aB
    d. Ab

10. What is the oxidation number of hydrogen in CaH_2?
    a. +1
    b. −1
    c. 0
    d. +2

11. Which hormone stimulates milk production in the breasts during lactation?
    a. norepinephrine
    b. antidiuretic hormone
    c. prolactin
    d. oxytocin

12. What is the typical result of mitosis in humans?
    a. two diploid cells
    b. two haploid cells
    c. four diploid cells
    d. four haploid cells

13. Which of the following does *not* exist as a diatomic molecule?
    a. boron
    b. fluorine
    c. oxygen
    d. nitrogen

14. Which of the following structures has the lowest blood pressure?
    a. arteries
    b. arteriole
    c. venule
    d. vein

15. How does water affect the temperature of a living thing?
    a. Water increases temperature.
    b. Water keeps temperature stable.
    c. Water decreases temperature.
    d. Water does not affect temperature.

16. What is another name for aqueous HI?
    a. hydroiodate acid
    b. hydrogen monoiodide
    c. hydrogen iodide
    d. hydriodic acid

17. Which of the heart chambers is the most muscular?
    a. left atrium
    b. right atrium
    c. left ventricle
    d. right ventricle

18. Which of the following is *not* a product of the Krebs cycle?
    a. carbon dioxide
    b. oxygen
    c. adenosine triphosphate (ATP)
    d. energy carriers

19. What is the name for the reactant that is entirely consumed by the reaction?
    a. limiting reactant
    b. reducing agent
    c. reaction intermediate
    d. reagent

20. Which part of the brain interprets sensory information?
    a. cerebrum
    b. hindbrain
    c. cerebellum
    d. medulla oblongata

21. What kind of bond connects sugar and phosphate in DNA?
    a. hydrogen
    b. ionic
    c. covalent
    d. overt

22. What is the mass (in grams) of 7.35 mol water?
    a. 10.7 g
    b. 18 g
    c. 132 g
    d. 180.6 g

23. Which of the following proteins is produced by cartilage?
    a. actin
    b. estrogen
    c. collagen
    d. myosin

24. How are lipids different than other organic molecules?
    a. They are indivisible.
    b. They are not water soluble.
    c. They contain zinc.
    d. They form long proteins.

25. Which of the following orbitals is the last to fill?
    a. 1s
    b. 3s
    c. 4p
    d. 6s

26. Which component of the nervous system is responsible for lowering the heart rate?
    a. central nervous system
    b. sympathetic nervous system
    c. parasympathetic nervous system
    d. distal nervous system

27. Which of the following is *not* a steroid?
    a. cholesterol
    b. estrogen
    c. testosterone
    d. hemoglobin

28. What is the name of the binary molecular compound NO_5?
    a. cnitro pentoxide
    b. ammonium pentoxide
    c. nitrogen pentoxide
    d. pentnitrogen oxide

29. In which of the following muscle types are the filaments arranged in a disorderly manner?
    a. cardiac
    b. smooth
    c. skeletal
    d. rough

30. Which hormone is produced by the pineal gland?
    a. insulin
    b. testosterone
    c. melatonin
    d. epinephrine

31. Make the following metric conversion: 5 decimeters = _____ decameters
    a. 0.5
    b. 0.05
    c. 50
    d. 500

32. Which of the data sets could be plotted on a pie chart?
   a. The total population of the top five largest U.S. cities.
   b. The incubation period of a penguin colony as it relates to hours of daylight.
   c. The distribution of weight among players of a football team.
   d. The percent of vegetation cover and precipitation rates in different national parks.

33. Which of the following processes uses electrical charges to separate substances?
   a. Spectrophotometry
   b. Chromatography
   c. Centrifugation
   d. Electrophoresis

34. When using a light microscope, how is the total magnification determined?
   a. By multiplying the ocular lens power times the objective being used.
   b. By looking at the objective you are using only.
   c. By looking at the ocular lens power only.
   d. By multiplying the objective you are using times two.

35. When undergoing a dissection in class, which of the following procedures is incorrect?
   a. Rinse the specimen before handling.
   b. Dispose of harmful chemicals according to district regulations.
   c. Decaying specimens are never permitted but unknown specimens are sometimes permitted.
   d. Students with open sores on their hands that cannot be covered should be excused from the dissection.

36. After a science laboratory exercise, some solutions remain unused and are left over. What should be done with these solutions?
   a. Dispose of the solutions according to local disposal procedures.
   b. Empty the solutions into the sink and rinse with warm water and soap.
   c. Ensure the solutions are secured in closed containers and throw away.
   d. Store the solutions in a secured, dry place for later use.

37. The volume of water in a bucket is 2.5 liters. When an object with an irregular shape and a mass of 40 grams is submerged in the water, the volume of the water is 4.5 liters. What is the density of the object?
   a. $\frac{1}{10}$ g/L
   b. 2 g/L
   c. 20 g/L
   d. 80 g/L

38. Which of the following represents a chemical change?
   a. Sublimation of water
   b. A spoiling apple
   c. Dissolution of salt in water
   d. Pulverized rock

39. The amount of potential energy an object has depends on all of the following except its:
    a. mass
    b. height above ground
    c. gravitational attraction
    d. temperature.

40. Elements on the periodic table are arranged into groups and periods and ordered according to:
    a. atomic number
    b. number of protons
    c. reactivity
    d. All of the above

41. The specific heat capacity of ice is half as much as that of liquid water. What is the result of this?
    a. It takes half the amount of energy to increase the temperature of a 1 kg sample of ice by 1°C than a 1 kg sample of water.
    b. It takes twice the amount of energy to increase the temperature of a 1 kg sample of ice by 1°C than a 1 kg sample of water.
    c. It takes a quarter the amount of energy to increase the temperature of a 1 kg sample of ice by 1°C than a 1 kg sample of water.
    d. It takes the same amount of energy to increase the temperature of a 1 kg sample of ice and a 1 kg sample of water by 1°C.

42. What happens to the temperature of a substance as it is changing phase from a liquid to a solid?
    a. Its temperature increases due to the absorption of latent heat.
    b. Its temperature decreases due to the heat of vaporization.
    c. Its temperature decreases due to the latent heat of fusion.
    d. Its temperature remains the same due to the latent heat of fusion.

43. A long nail is heated at one end. After a few seconds, the other end of the nail becomes equally hot. What type of heat transfer does this represent?
    a. Radiation
    b. Conduction
    c. Convection
    d. Entropy

44. Which of the following statements about heat transfer is not true?
    a. As the energy of a system changes, its thermal energy must change or work must be done.
    b. Heat transfer from a warmer object to a cooler object can occur spontaneously.
    c. Heat transfer can never occur from a cooler object to a warmer object.
    d. If two objects reach the same temperature, energy is no longer available for work.

45. The measure of energy within a system is called _____.
    a. temperature
    b. heat
    c. entropy
    d. thermodynamics

46. Which of the following is true of an isotope?
    a. It has a different number of protons than its element.
    b. It has a different number of electrons than its element.
    c. It has a different charge as compared to its element.
    d. It has a different number of neutrons than its element.

47. If an atom's outer shell is filled, what must be true?
    a. It reacts with other atoms through chemical reactions.
    b. It exchanges electrons to form bonds with other atoms.
    c. It has 32 electrons in its outer shell.
    d. It is a stable atom.

48. Which type of nuclear process features atomic nuclei splitting apart to form smaller nuclei?
    a. Fission
    b. Fusion
    c. Decay
    d. Ionization

49. Electrons with greater amounts of energy are found _____ the nucleus than electrons with less energy.
    a. closer to
    b. farther from
    c. more often inside
    d. more randomly around

50. The process whereby a radioactive element releases energy slowly over a long period of time to lower its energy and become more stable is best described as _____.
    a. combustion
    b. fission
    c. fusion
    d. decay

51. Which of the following is a type of simple machine?
    a. A bicycle
    b. A pair of scissors
    c. A screw
    d. A shovel

52. In which of the following scenarios is work not applied to the object?
    a. Mario moves a book from the floor to the top shelf.
    b. A book drops off the shelf and falls to the floor.
    c. Mario pushes a box of books across the room.
    d. Mario balances a book on his head and walks across the room.

53. A ball is resting on the front end of a boat. The boat is moving straight forwards toward a dock. According to Newton's first law of motion, when the front of the boat hits the dock, how will the ball's motion change?
   a. The ball will remain at rest.
   b. The ball will move backwards.
   c. The ball will move forwards.
   d. The ball will move sideways.

54. What two things are required for circular motion to occur?
   a. Acceleration and centripetal force
   b. Acceleration and gravitational force
   c. Constant speed and centripetal force
   d. Constant speed and gravitational force

55. According to Bernoulli's Principle, where will a gas flowing through a pipe exert the least amount of pressure?
   a. Where the pipe is widest
   b. Where the pipe is narrowest
   c. Where its velocity is lowest
   d. Where its kinetic energy is lowest

56. If a glass rod is rubbed with a cloth made of polyester, what will the resulting charge be on each material?
   a. The charge on the glass rod is positive and the charge on the cloth is negative.
   b. The charge on the glass rod is negative and the charge on the cloth is positive.
   c. The charge on the glass rod is neutral and the charge on the cloth is positive.
   d. The charge on the glass rod and the cloth both become neutral.

57. According to Ohm's Law, how are voltage and current related in an electrical circuit?
   a. Voltage and current are inversely proportional to one another.
   b. Voltage and current are directly proportional to one another.
   c. Voltage acts to oppose the current along an electrical circuit.
   d. Voltage acts to decrease the current along an electrical circuit.

58. A material becomes magnetic when the individual electrons of an atom _____, allowing their magnetic fields to add together.
   a. spin in pairs in opposite directions
   b. spin in pairs in the same direction
   c. spin unpaired
   d. stop spinning

59. In a parallel circuit, there are three paths: A, B and C. Path A has a resistance of 10 ohms, path B a resistance of 5 ohms and part C a resistance of 2 ohms. How do the voltage and current change for each path?
   a. Voltage and current are kept the same in each path.
   b. Voltage is greatest in path A and current is greatest in path C.
   c. Voltage is lowest in path C and current is greatest in path C.
   d. Voltage is the same for each path and current is greatest in path C.

60. A rock concert is taking place outdoors. In which of the following conditions will their sound travel the farthest?
    a. High temperature and low humidity
    b. High temperature and humidity
    c. Low temperature and humidity
    d. Low temperature and high humidity

Answers and Explanations

Academic Aptitude

Verbal

1. A: Expand means get bigger. Contract, shrink, diminish, and lessen mean get smaller.

2. B: Adore means love. Abhor, despise, hate, and deplore mean the opposite.

3. C: Original means new or unfamiliar, the opposite of trite, cliché, overused, and commonplace.

4. D: To cooperate is to agree or get along; to bicker, argue, quarrel, or disagree are opposites.

5. E: Pandemonium, chaos, excitement, and disarray are wild, disordered states; harmony is not.

6. B: Gleeful means joyful, delighted, and happy. Somber, serious, sad, and gloomy are opposites.

7. C: Apprehension, trepidation, dread, and anxiety are worried states; optimism or hope is not.

8. D: Dismal, dreary, bleak, and depressing are synonyms; cheery is their antonym/opposite.

9. A: Fortunate means lucky. Hapless, unlucky, tragic, and doomed all mean the opposite.

10. C: To disperse is to thin (out), dissipate, or scatter; to collect is to gather/come together.

11. C: Aware is knowledgeable/informed; oblivious, clueless, heedless, and ignorant are opposites.

12. D: Distraught means very anxious, alarmed, agitated, or distracted; tranquil is peaceful, an antonym.

13. E: Bedlam, confusion, havoc, and uproar are like disorganization/disorder; order is the opposite.

14. B: Clear means easily understood. The other choices are all antonyms.

15. A: Invite is to ask or encourage; avert means to prevent; evade and elude mean to escape.

16. A: Unique is unusual/singular/one-of-a-kind; mundane, pedestrian, and quotidian mean ordinary.

17. C: Perpetual is always, constant, ceaseless, running, or continual; occasional is once in a while.

18. B: Vexing is irritating, annoying, or aggravating. Gratifying means pleasing, the opposite.

19. D: Sagacious means wise, knowing, or astute. Ignorant means unknowing, the opposite.

20. E: Audacious means bold, brash, forward, or rude. Humble is a near opposite, meaning modest.

21. A: Deriding is mocking or scorning. Approving, praising, favoring, and commending are antonyms.

22. E: Stealthy is sneaky, secretive, sly, or furtive; transparent is open, clear, or obvious, the opposite.

23. C: Impudent means sassy, rude, impertinent, or disrespectful; respectful means the opposite.

24. D: Blissful, blithe, jubilant, and jocund mean delighted/joyful/happy; aggrieved means sad/unhappy.

25. B: Gaunt means haggard, wasted, or skinny. Plump means chubby, fat, or fleshy, the opposite.

26. A: Unassuming is modest/humble; haughty, superior, lofty, and presumptuous are proud/arrogant.

27. B: Reverent is religious; blasphemous, profane, impious, and sacrilegious are disrespecting religion.

28. C: A heretic, renegade, defector, or dissident opposes accepted beliefs; believers do not.

29. B: Cynical means mistrustful, skeptical, suspicious, negative, or pessimistic; trusting is the opposite.

30. D: Agape means openmouthed, anticipating eagerly, or agog; unmoved has the opposite meaning.

Arithmetic

1. D: This is a simple addition problem. Start with the ones column (on the right). Add the figures 6+1, 3+0, 2+3 to get the answer 537.

2. C: This is a simple addition problem with carrying. Start with the ones column and add 7+4, write down the 1 and add the 1 to the digits in the tens column. Now add 0+6+1. Write down the 7. Now add 3+8 and write down the 1. Add the 1 to the thousands column. Add 4+1+1 and write the 6 to get the answer 6171.

3. B: Simply substitute the given values for *a* and *b* and perform the required operations.

4. A: This is a subtraction problem which involves borrowing. Start with the ones column. Since 7 can't be subtracted from 6, borrow ten from the tens column. Cross out the 5 and make it a 4. Now subtract 7 from 16. Write down 9. Move to the tens column Since 6 can't be subtracted from 4, borrow ten from the hundreds column. Cross out the 3 and make it a 2.   14-6 = 8. Now subtract 1 from 2 and write down 1 to get 189.

5. B: This is a subtraction problem which also involves borrowing. Start with the ones column. Since 7 can't be subtracted from 6, borrow ten from the tens column. Cross out the 0 and make it a 9. Cross out the 2 in the hundreds column and make it a 2. Now subtract 7 from 16. Write down 9.

Move to the tens column. Subtract 8 from 9 and write down 1. Move to the hundreds column. Since you can't subtract 4 from 3, borrow ten from the thousands column. Cross out the 5 and make it a 4. 12-4= 8. Now subtract 3 from 4 and write down 1 to get 1819.

6. C: This problem is solved by finding x in this equation: $34/80 = x/100$.

7. A: This is a multiplication problem with 0. Start with the 7 in 17 and multiply it by each of the digits at the top 7 x 7. Write down the 9 and place the 4 in the tens column. 7 x 0 is 0. Add the 4. 7 x 7 is 49. The top line will read 4949. Now multiply 1 by 7. Write down the 7. 1 x 0 is 0 and 1 x 7 is 7. The bottom line will read 707. Add these together with the 7 in the tens column and the answer will be 12,019.

8. A: This is a simple division problem. Divide the 7 into 9. It goes in 1 time. Write 1 above the 9 and subtract 7 from 9 to get 2. Bring down the 1 and place it beside the 2. Divide 7 into 21. It goes in 3 times. Divide 7 into 7. It goes 1 time.

9. D: To solve this problem, work backwards. That is, perform FOIL on each answer choice until you derive the original expression.

10. A: To change this fraction into a decimal, divide 100 into 38. 100 goes into 38 .38 times.

11. C: This is a simple addition problem. Line up the decimals so that they are all in the same place in the equation, and see that there is a 6 by itself in the hundredths column. Then add the tenths column: 8+3to get 11. Write down the 1 and carry the 1. Add the ones column: 6+1 plus the carried 1. Write down 8. Then write down the 1.

12. A: A set of six numbers with an average of 4 must have a collective sum of 24. The two numbers that average 2 will add up to 4, so the remaining numbers must add up to 20. The average of these four numbers can be calculated: 20/4 = 5.

13. C: Count from the 3: tenths, hundredths, thousandths.

14. A: This is a simple subtraction problem with decimals. Line up the decimals and subtract 9 from 8. Since this can't be done, borrow 10 from the 5. Cross out the 5 and make it 4. Now subtract 9 from 18 to get 9. Subtract 3 from 4 and get 1. Place the decimal point before the 1.

15. D: Simple Multiplication.

16. A: To add fractions, ensure that the denominator (the number on the bottom) is the same. Since it is not, change them both to 56ths. 1/8 equals 7/56. 3/7 equals 24/56. Now add the whole numbers: 3+6 = 9 and the fractions 31/56.

17. C: To subtract fractions, ensure that the denominator (the number on the bottom) is the same. Since it is not, change them both to 14ths. 17 equals 2/14. 1/2 equals 7/14. The equation now looks like this: $4\frac{3}{14} - 2\frac{7}{14}$. Change the 4 to 3 and add 14 to the numerator (the top number) so that the fractions can be subtracted. The equation now looks like this: $3\frac{16}{14} - 2\frac{97}{14}$. Subtract: $1\frac{9}{14}$

18. A: To multiply mixed numbers, first create improper fractions. Multiply the whole number by the denominator, and then add the numerator. $1\frac{1}{4}$ becomes $\frac{5}{4}$.

The problem will look like this: $\frac{5}{4} \times \frac{17}{15} \times \frac{5}{3} = \frac{425}{60} = 7\frac{1}{12}$

19. C: There are 12 inches in a foot and 3 feet in a yard. Four and a half yards is equal to 162 inches. To determine the number of 3-inche segments, divide 162 by 3.

20. C: Divide the numerator and denominator by 14.

21. A: Write .36, and then move the decimal two places. Add the percent sign.

22. C: 10% of 900 are 90. Multiply 90 by 4 to find 40%.

23. A: If it takes 3 people 3 1/3 days to do the job, then it would take one person 10 days: $3 \times 3\frac{1}{3} = 10$. Thus, it would take 2 people 5 days, and one day of work for two people would complete 1/5 of the job.

24. A: Divide 40 by 8 to get 5. Multiply 5 by 3 to get 15.

25. B: Rewrite the problem as 0.06*25 and solve.

26. D: Divide 4 by 16 (not 16 by 4)

27. C: Since 4 is the same as 2^2, $4^6 = 2^{12}$. When dividing exponents with the same base, simply subtract the exponent in the denominator from the exponent in the numerator.

28. D: To solve, rewrite the percent as a fraction: $\frac{30}{100}$. Then reduce the fraction.

29. C: To change a percent to a decimal, remove the percent sign and move the decimal two spaces to the left.

30. A: To solve, add 6 a and 2a, then subtract 4a.

Nonverbal

1. A: The first figure has a circle inside the rectangle; in the second figure, the inner shape is removed. The third figure is a circle with a rectangular inner shape. (A) is a circle like the third figure, with the inner shape removed as it is in the second figure.

2. B: The first figure is a larger rectangle, and the second figure is a smaller rectangle. The third figure is a larger circle, and (B) is a smaller circle.

3. C: The first figure is a circle with a smaller circle inside; the second figure is a rectangle with a smaller rectangle inside. The third figure is like the smaller inner circle from the first figure without the larger outer circle, and (C) is like the smaller rectangle from the second figure without the larger outer rectangle.

4. D: The first figure is a rectangle, and the second, a triangle, is one half diagonally of the first rectangle. The third figure is a circle, and (D) is one half diagonally of the circle.

5. E: Of the choices given, the corner section (E) of the rectangle in the third figure is most like the semicircular section shown in the second figure of the ring/circle shown in the first figure.

6. D: The triangle in the first figure is inverted (turned upside down) in the second figure. The semicircular shape in the third figure is also inverted in (D).

7. C: The first figure is a star with 4 points and the second figure is a star with 5 points. The third figure is a star with 6 points. Continuing the pattern of adding 1 point, (C) is a star with 7 points.

8. B: The first figure is the right half of a circle, and the second figure is a full circle. The third figure is the right half of a diamond, and (B) is a full diamond.

9. A: The first two figures are both rectangles; the first contains vertical stripes, and the second contains horizontal stripes. The third figure is a circle containing vertical stripes. Therefore, the circle containing horizontal stripes in (A) repeats the pattern.

10. B: The first diamond is clear, and the second is filled with a diamond-checked design. The third figure, a circle, is clear like the first diamond; therefore, the circle filled with the diamond-checked design in (B) follows the pattern.

11. C: The first figure is a small sunburst; the second figure is a larger sunburst. The third figure is a small smiley face, so the larger smiley face in (C) creates a matching relationship.

12. D: The first figure is a right-angled shape with an arrow point on one end; the second figure is a right-angled shape with arrow points on both ends. The third figure is a straight shape with an arrow point on one end, so the straight shape with arrow points on both ends (D) matches the relationship.

13. C: The first figure is like a block equal sign with a diagonal slash; the second figure is a ring/circle, also with a diagonal slash. The third figure is like the first equal sign, but with no slash. Therefore the ring with no slash (C) is most like the third figure.

14. D: The first figure is a circle filled with a checkerboard design, and the second circle is clear. The third figure is a rectangle filled with the checkerboard design, so the clear rectangle (D) corresponds.

15. E: In the first figure, two triangles are joined point to point; in the second, two hearts are joined, also point to point. In the third figure, the triangles are joined at their broader bases rather than their points; the two hearts in (E) are also joined at their broader tops rather than their points.

16. B: The first figure is a curve with an arrow pointing up; the second is a curve with an arrow pointing down. The third figure is straight with an arrow pointing up; therefore, the straight figure with an arrow pointing down (B) matches the relationship.

17. A: The first figure is a triangle filled with a zigzag design; the second is a triangle filled with a grid design. The third figure is a circle filled with a zigzag design; therefore, the circle filled with a grid design (A) shows the same relationship.

18. E: The heart in the first figure is inverted in the second figure. The third figure is a triangle; this shape is inverted in (E) the same way that the heart is.

19. E: The first figure has two crescent shapes with their points facing each other; in the second figure, the points face away. The third figure has a pair of angular brackets, facing each other like the first pair of crescents. Therefore, the pair of angular brackets facing away from each other (E) matches the second pair of crescents.

20. B: The first figure, a circle, has been elongated and narrowed into a long, thin oval in the second figure. The third figure, a diamond, is likewise made longer and thinner in (B).

21. A: The first diamond has diagonal stripes going from the lower left to the upper right; the second diamond has diagonal stripes going from the upper left to the lower right. The third figure is a circle with diagonal stripes matching those in the first diamond; therefore, the circle with diagonal stripes matching those in the second diamond follows the pattern.

22. C: The first two figures point to the right, and they would dovetail if put together. The third figure also points to the right but is rounded rather than angled; the rounded shape, also pointing right in (C), would also dovetail with the third figure if they were put together.

23. E: The first two lines have the same right angles, but the first one has arrows at both ends, pointing up and down; the second has an arrow on only one end, pointing down. The third figure is straight, with arrows at both ends. Therefore, the straight figure with an arrow on only one end pointing down (E) relates to the third figure the same way.

24. D: The first line has two right-angled bends, with one arrow at the top; the second line has the same angles, but it has arrows at both top and bottom. The third figure is curved, with one arrow at the top, so the curved line with arrows at both top and bottom (D) follows the same relationship.

25. D: The first figure has four arrow points, and the second has three. The third figure also has three arrow points. The figure with two arrow points (D) continues the pattern of subtracting one arrow point. (4 : 3 is as 3 : 2.)

26. C: The first figure is a circle with two progressively smaller circles inside. The second figure is like the first but with the smallest circle removed. The third figure is a rectangle with two progressively smaller rectangles inside, so the rectangle missing the smallest inner rectangle (C) repeats the pattern.

27. B: The first figure is a diamond with a smaller diamond inside. The second figure is like the first, but with a third, even smaller diamond inside of the others. The third figure is a circle with a smaller circle inside. Therefore, the circle containing two smaller circles (B) follows the same relationship.

28. E: The second figure, a crescent, is a section of the first figure, a circle. The third figure is a rectangle, and the corner piece (E) is correspondingly a section of it.

29. A: The second shape is the first shape, inverted. The third shape is also inverted in choice (A).

30. A: The first shape is the top half of the second shape. Likewise, the third shape is the top half of the shape in (A).

Spelling

1. A: separate

2. B: nuclear

3. C: familiar

4. A: sacrilegious

5. C: agitated

6. B: oriented

7. C: indispensable

8. A: similar

9. B: attitude

10. B: abbreviate

11. A: absorb

12. C: accumulate

13. C: aerial

14. A: comedian

15. B: asphalt

16. B: forcible

17. C: anecdote

18. A: flexible

19. A: defendant

20. C: plaintiff

21. B: idiosyncrasy

22. A: hazardous

23. B: horrific

24. C: handsome

25. A: liaison

26. B: galaxy

27. A: attorneys

28. C: asterisk

29. C: equilibrium

30. A: brilliance

31. B: blanch.

32. A: ecstasy

33. B: depreciate

34. C: turpitude

35. B: opposite

36. C: tyranny

37. A: schism

38. C: schedule

39. A: incandescent

40. B: terrific

41. B: homogenize

42. A: sieve

43. C: truly

44. A: sincerely

45. B: transient

46. A: sedition

47. C: thieves

48. B: vengeance

49. B: nylon

50. C: unacceptable

51. A: deficit

52. B: disapproval

53. A: diffidence

54. C: picnicking

55. C: oregano

56. B: bachelor

57. A: indelible

58. B: diurnal

59. A: impatience

60. C: parliament

Reading Comprehension

1. B: Paragraph 1 states the parents married before World War II, and everything that follows occurs after that.

2. C: The last sentence of the first paragraph identifies Nana as what the children called Marian's mother, who was therefore their grandmother. It also identifies Fluffy as the cat's name (B).

3. D: Sentence #6 of 8 in paragraph 2 states that Marian had contracted poison oak while petting the Irish setter Katie, who had rubbed against Marian's bare legs.

4. A: Sentence #4 of paragraph 1 states that the couple lived with Marian's widowed mother. The last sentence of this paragraph also states that the children called Marian's mother Nana.

5. A: Sentence #3 of paragraph 1 says Bernard was in the Army. Sentence #4 refers to his tour of duty. This means the term a soldier serves in the military forces.

6. C: Paragraph 3 describes the family hearing Fluffy meow during dinner (B), but this was not how they discovered where he had been; it was by seeing him go back up the chimney where he had been hiding all along.

7. D: Paragraph 3 identifies the chimney as a cool place (B) to escape from all the commotion (C), so these are both correct. Cats generally tend to hide, but when frightened, not always (A).

8. C: Sentence 1 of paragraph 4 says cats hate changes in their environment (A), and identifies the noise and confusion of moving (B). The beginning of this sentence describes the cat's need for safety and seclusion/privacy (D). Paragraph 2 identifies a dog in the neighborhood (C), but not in the house; the passage states Fluffy was never outdoors. Fluffy could have smelled the dog's scent on Marian, who had petted her, and also from a distance; but considering the more direct factors of (A), (B), and (D), this is the *least* likely reason the cat found moving day traumatic.

- 133 -

9. C: The penultimate sentence of the final paragraph describes Fluffy doing (A), (B), and (D), but never mentions his climbing drapes in Lewis's room (C).

10. D: The main focus of the passage is how the family "lost" and then found their pet while moving. The other choices are all details included in the story rather than its main topic.

11. C: The earliest use of this title and lyric identified in this passage were by Al Dubin and Harry Warren in 1933. Billie Joe Armstrong (A) used it in 2004. Tony Bennett and Sting (B) recorded a duet covering the Dubin and Warren original in 2006. Gottfried Helnwein (D) gave his painting this title in 1984.

12. D: The passage states that Hopper named his famous painting *Nighthawks. Boulevard of Broken Dreams* (A) was the name of Gottfried Helnwein's painting, which was a parody of Hopper's *Nighthawks. American Idiot* (B) was the title of Green Day's 2004 album that included their original song, inspired by Helnwein's painting and also entitled *Boulevard of Broken Dreams. Strange Wine* (C) was the title of Harlan Ellison's 1978 collection of science fiction short stories, which included his story entitled *Boulevard of Broken Dreams.*

13. A: The passage says Constance Bennett sang this song in the 1934 movie. It says later that Tony Bennett and Sting (B) covered it in a duet in 2006. It identifies a different song with the same title being (written and) sung by Billie Joe (Armstrong) and Green Day (C) in 2004. And it states that Juan García Esquivel (D) recorded a song with this title in 1958.

14. B: The passage states that Hopper created his original painting using oils, and that Helnwein painted his parody of Hopper's work using watercolors.

15. D: The passage quotes these lyrics, identifying them as from the Green Day song written by Billie Joe Armstrong. The passage also quotes lyrics from the 1933 Dubin (A) and Warren (B) song, including "Here is where you'll always find me/Always walking up and down...." But the earlier song is never quoted to (and does not in fact) include "I walk alone, I walk alone" as Armstrong's song does. Constance Bennett (C) sang the older song in the movie *Moulin Rouge* but did not write it.

16. D: None of these celebrities is portrayed in Hopper's painting: the passage describes the four people in Hopper's painting as "anonymous." Dean (A), Presley (B), Monroe (C), and Humphrey Bogart are all depicted in Gottfried Helnwein's painting, a later parody of Hopper's work.

17. C: The passage indicates that Ellison published a short story with this title in 1978. It identifies Alexander's biography of Dean (A) as published in 1994. It states that Deitch's graphic novel (B) was published in 2002. And it identifies the E! TV network as airing a documentary series with this title (D) in 2007.

18. B: The passage reports that Green Day's song was inspired by Gottfried Helnwein's parody painting entitled *Boulevard of Broken Dreams.* The famous painting by Edward Hopper (A) was entitled *Nighthawks* and not named as an inspiration for Green Day's song. Neither is the 1933 song (C) of the same title, which was sung in the 1934 movie *Moulin Rouge* (D), also not Green Day's source.

19. A: This passage includes paintings, songs, albums, movies, books, and a TV series using the title. It identifies both single songs and albums (B); a science fiction book and a graphic novel (C); and a documentary series on TV (D).

20. A: The passage dates Helnwein's painting with the celebrities to 1984. It says the celebrities pictured had all died young between 1955 and 1977.* Thus they were not still alive [(C), (D)]. Since Helnwein made the painting seven years after the latest death and 29 years after the earliest one, they had not just recently died (B). *(James Dean died in 1955; Humphrey Bogart in 1957; Marilyn Monroe in 1962; and Elvis Presley in 1977.)

21. D: The passage indicates (first paragraph) that imidacloprid is chemically related to nicotine, but never says it is used as a nicotine substitute. It does say this pesticide is used for killing fleas on pets (A), killing garden pests (B), and protecting farm crops (C).

22. D: Both A and C. The passage explains that imidacloprid gets into corn kernels (A), and also that it is present in corn syrup, which people ingest (C). It never says they inhale it from the air (B).

23. C: Both. The passage states that Dr. Lu worked at Emory University (A) in 2006 and at Harvard University (B) at its School of Public Health in 2010. Hence, neither (D) is false.

24. C: Dr. Lu's 2010 experiment proved that feeding bees H-F corn syrup dosed with imidacloprid killed them. Therefore, even if it is not the sole cause of bee colony collapse disorder, the cause is certainly associated with the use of this pesticide. Hence, while not everything is known, it is not still a complete mystery (A). The passage does not say there are factors too numerous to mention (B). Bee colony collapse disorder is not found to be caused by the corn syrup (D) itself but the pesticide in it.

25. B: The passage explains that imidacloprid kills insects by disrupting their brain neurons' uptake of acetylcholine, not destroying the neurons (A). Acetylcholine is identified as necessary for muscles to work, not as toxic (C). Since the mechanism of imidacloprid (a neurotoxin) is described as disrupting neuronal acetylcholine uptake, it is not true that the mechanism is unknown (D).

26. B: The passage relates that in Lu's 2006 study, the organophosphate (chemicals in pesticides) residues in school children's urine disappeared right away when the children were switched to organic (pesticide-free) diets. These residues did not persist despite the dietary change (A). There is nothing about school children dying from high-fructose corn syrup (C). Beehive populations (D) were not included in Lu's 2006 experiment; he studied bees in 2010. [Even in Lu's 2010 experiment, the bees did not die from the corn syrup (D), but from the pesticide he added to it.]

27. A: All but one of the beehive populations fed corn syrup laced with imidacloprid died in Lu's experiment. The passage indicates that he conducted this study in the summer, not winter (B) [which is when beehives are commonly fed corn syrup]; and it was not the syrup itself [also (B)] but the pesticide that killed them. No school children [(C), (D)] participated in Lu's 2010 experiment.

28. A: The passage states that Dr. Lu has concluded that even low dosages of pesticides can cause human health problems, not only very high doses (B). While Lu found that pesticides in corn syrup kills bees, the passage never says he concluded it does not affect humans (C), but rather that it can. Lu did not conclude that imidacloprid use on crops should be immediately banned (D); he concluded, rather, that without sufficient human data that have not yet been collected, its use could continue to be approved for 20–30 years longer.

- 135 -

29. C: The passage indicates that chemical residues in foods *are* monitored (A), but *not* in *all* foods (B); for example, not in H-F corn syrup. It also states this is because the syrup itself is *not* directly sold to consumers (D).

30. B: The passage refers to Dr. Lu's statement that without plenty of human data, imidacloprid can be approved for crop use for 20–30 years longer; hence he did not say it will be discontinued very soon (A). The passage includes the information that Dr. Lu has found even very low levels of imidacloprid harms bees (C). It also indicates that Lu said *no* data about imidacloprid's effects on humans have been gathered (D). As the passage reports, this lack of human data is why Lu says the chemical's use on crops may continue for 20–30 more years.

Natural Science

1. D: The name for a substance that stimulates the production of antibodies is an *antigen*. An antigen is any substance perceived by the immune system as dangerous. When the body senses an antigen, it produces an antibody. *Collagen* is one of the components of bone, tendon, and cartilage. It is a spongy protein that can be turned into gelatin by boiling. *Hemoglobin* is the part of red blood cells that carries oxygen. In order for the blood to carry enough oxygen to the cells of the body, there has to be a sufficient amount of hemoglobin. *Lymph* is a near-transparent fluid that performs a number of functions in the body: It removes bacteria from tissues, replaces lymphocytes in the blood, and moves fat away from the small intestine. Lymph contains white blood cells. As you can see, some of the questions in the vocabulary section will require technical knowledge.

2. D: The cellular hierarchy starts with the cell, the simplest structure, and progresses to organisms, the most complex structures.

3. B: A hypertonic solution is a solution with a higher particle concentration than in the cell, and consequently lower water content than in the cell. Water moves from the cell to the solution, causing the cell to experience water loss and shrink.

4. A: The immune system consists of the lymphatic system, spleen, tonsils, thymus and bone marrow.

5. D: The rate at which a chemical reaction occurs does not depend on the amount of mass lost, since the law of conservation of mass (or matter) states that in a chemical reaction there is no loss of mass.

6. B: Boyle's law states that for a constant mass and temperature, pressure and volume are related inversely to one another: PV = c, where c = constant.

7. C: Prokaryotic cells are simpler cells that do not have membrane-bound organelles, whereas eukaryotic cells have several membrane-bound organelles.

8. A: A ribosome is a structure of eukaryotic cells that makes proteins.

9. B: It is impossible for an *AaBb* organism to have the *aa* combination in the gametes. It is impossible for each letter to be used more than one time, so it would be impossible for the

- 136 -

lowercase *a* to appear twice in the gametes. It would be possible, however, for *Aa* to appear in the gametes, since there is one uppercase *A* and one lowercase *a*. Gametes are the cells involved in sexual reproduction. They are germ cells.

10. B: The oxidation number of the hydrogen in CaH_2 is −1. The oxidation number is the positive or negative charge of a monoatomic ion. In other words, the oxidation number is the numerical charge on an ion. An ion is a charged version of an element. Oxidation number is often referred to as oxidation state. Oxidation number is sometimes used to describe the number of electrons that must be added or removed from an atom in order to convert the atom to its elemental form.

11. C: *Prolactin* stimulates the production of breast milk during lactation. *Norepinephrine* is a hormone and neurotransmitter secreted by the adrenal gland that regulates heart rate, blood pressure, and blood sugar. *Antidiuretic hormone* is produced by the hypothalamus and secreted by the pituitary gland. It regulates the concentration of urine and triggers the contractions of the arteries and capillaries. *Oxytocin* is a hormone secreted by the pituitary gland that makes it easier to eject milk from the breast and manages the contractions of the uterus during labor.

12. A: The typical result of mitosis in humans is two diploid cells. *Mitosis* is the division of a body cell into two daughter cells. Each of the two produced cells has the same set of chromosomes as the parent. A diploid cell contains both sets of homologous chromosomes. A haploid cell contains only one set of chromosomes, which means that it only has a single set of genes.

13. A: Boron does not exist as a diatomic molecule. The other possible answer choices, fluorine, oxygen, and nitrogen, all exist as diatomic molecules. A diatomic molecule always appears in nature as a pair: The word *diatomic* means "having two atoms." With the exception of astatine, all of the halogens are diatomic. Chemistry students often use the mnemonic BrINClHOF (pronounced "brinkelhoff") to remember all of the diatomic elements: bromine, iodine, nitrogen, chlorine, hydrogen, oxygen, and fluorine. Note that not all of these diatomic elements are halogens.

14. D: Of the given structures, veins have the lowest blood pressure. *Veins* carry oxygen-poor blood from the outlying parts of the body to the heart. An *artery* carries oxygen-rich blood from the heart to the peripheral parts of the body. An *arteriole* extends from an artery to a capillary. A *venule* is a tiny vein that extends from a capillary to a larger vein.

15. B: Water stabilizes the temperature of living things. The ability of warm-blooded animals, including human beings, to maintain a constant internal temperature is known as *homeostasis*. Homeostasis depends on the presence of water in the body. Water tends to minimize changes in temperature because it takes a while to heat up or cool down. When the human body gets warm, the blood vessels dilate and blood moves away from the torso and toward the extremities. When the body gets cold, blood concentrates in the torso. This is the reason why hands and feet tend to get especially cold in cold weather.

16. D: Hydriodic acid is another name for aqueous HI. In an aqueous solution, the solvent is water. Hydriodic acid is a polyatomic ion, meaning that it is composed of two or more elements. When this solution has an increased amount of oxygen, the -*ate* suffix on the first word is converted to -*ic*.

17. C: Of the four heart chambers, the left ventricle is the most muscular. When it contracts, it pushes blood out to the organs and extremities of the body. The right ventricle pushes blood into the lungs. The atria, on the other hand, receive blood from the outlying parts of the body and transport it into the ventricles. The basic process works as follows: Oxygen-poor blood fills the right

atrium and is pumped into the right ventricle, from which it is pumped into the pulmonary artery and on to the lungs. In the lungs, this blood is oxygenated. The blood then reenters the heart at the left atrium, which when full pumps into the left ventricle. When the left ventricle is full, blood is pushed into the aorta and on to the organs and extremities of the body.

18. B: Oxygen is not one of the products of the Krebs cycle. The *Krebs cycle* is the second stage of cellular respiration. In this stage, a sequence of reactions converts pyruvic acid into carbon dioxide. This stage of cellular respiration produces the phosphate compounds that provide most of the energy for the cell. The Krebs cycle is also known as the citric acid cycle or the tricarboxylic acid cycle.

19. A: A limiting reactant is entirely used up by the chemical reaction. Limiting reactants control the extent of the reaction and determine the quantity of the product. A reducing agent is a substance that reduces the amount of another substance by losing electrons. A reagent is any substance used in a chemical reaction. Some of the most common reagents in the laboratory are sodium hydroxide and hydrochloric acid. The behavior and properties of these substances are known, so they can be effectively used to produce predictable reactions in an experiment.

20. A: The *cerebrum* is the part of the brain that interprets sensory information. It is the largest part of the brain. The cerebrum is divided into two hemispheres, connected by a thin band of tissue called the corpus callosum. The *cerebellum* is positioned at the back of the head, between the brain stem and the cerebrum. It controls both voluntary and involuntary movements. The *medulla oblongata* forms the base of the brain. This part of the brain is responsible for blood flow and breathing, among other things.

21. C: The sugar and phosphate in DNA are connected by covalent bonds. A *covalent bond* is formed when atoms share electrons. It is very common for atoms to share pairs of electrons. An *ionic bond* is created when one or more electrons are transferred between atoms. *Ionic bonds*, also known as *electrovalent bonds*, are formed between ions with opposite charges. There is no such thing as an *overt bond* in chemistry.

22. C: The mass of 7.35 mol water is 132 grams. You should be able to find the mass of various chemical compounds when you are given the number of mols. The information required to perform this function is included on the periodic table. To solve this problem, find the molecular mass of water by finding the respective weights of hydrogen and oxygen. Remember that water contains two hydrogen molecules and one oxygen molecule. The molecular mass of hydrogen is roughly 1, and the molecular mass of oxygen is roughly 16. A molecule of water, then, has approximately 18 grams of mass. Multiply this by 7.35 mol, and you will obtain the answer 132.3, which is closest to answer choice C.

23. C: *Collagen* is the protein produced by cartilage. Bone, tendon, and cartilage are all mainly composed of collagen. *Actin* and *myosin* are the proteins responsible for muscle contractions. Actin makes up the thinner fibers in muscle tissue, while myosin makes up the thicker fibers. Myosin is the most numerous cell protein in human muscle. *Estrogen* is one of the steroid hormones produced mainly by the ovaries. Estrogen motivates the menstrual cycle and the development of female sex characteristics.

24. B: Unlike other organic molecules, lipids are not water soluble. Lipids are typically composed of carbon and hydrogen. Three common types of lipid are fats, waxes, and oils. Indeed, lipids usually feel oily when you touch them. All living cells are primarily composed of lipids, carbohydrates, and

proteins. Some examples of fats are lard, corn oil, and butter. Some examples of waxes are beeswax and carnauba wax. Some examples of steroids are cholesterol and ergosterol.

25. D: Of these orbitals, the last to fill is 6s. Orbitals fill in the following order: 1s, 2s, 2p, 3s, 3p, 4s, 3d, 4p, 5s, 4d, 5p, 6s, 4f, 5d, 6p, 7s, 5f, 6d, and 7p. The number is the orbital number, and the letter is the sublevel identification. Sublevel s has one orbital and can hold a maximum of two electrons. Sublevel p has three orbitals and can hold a maximum of six electrons. Sublevel d has five orbitals and can hold a maximum of 10 electrons. Sublevel f has seven orbitals and can hold a maximum of 14 electrons.

26. C: The parasympathetic nervous system is responsible for lowering the heart rate. It slows down the heart rate, dilates the blood vessels, and increases the secretions of the digestive system. The central nervous system is composed of the brain and the spinal cord. The sympathetic nervous system is a part of the autonomic nervous system; its role is to oppose the actions taken by the parasympathetic nervous system. So, the sympathetic nervous system accelerates the heart, contracts the blood vessels, and decreases the secretions of the digestive system.

27. D: *Hemoglobin* is not a steroid. It is a protein that helps to move oxygen from the lungs to the various body tissues. Steroids can be either synthetic chemicals used to reduce swelling and inflammation or sex hormones produced by the body. *Cholesterol* is the most abundant steroid in the human body. It is necessary for the creation of bile, though it can be dangerous if the levels in the body become too high. *Estrogen* is a female steroid produced by the ovaries (in females), testes (in males), placenta, and adrenal cortex. It contributes to adolescent sexual development, menstruation, mood, lactation, and aging. *Testosterone* is the main hormone produced by the testes; it is responsible for the development of adult male sex characteristics.

28. C: Nitrogen pentoxide is the name of the binary molecular compound NO_5. The format given in answer choice C is appropriate when dealing with two nonmetals. A prefix is used to denote the number of atoms of each element. Note that when there are seven atoms of a given element, the prefix *hepta-* is used instead of the usual *septa-*. Also, when the first atom in this kind of binary molecular compound is single, it does not need to be given the prefix *mono-*.

29. B: Smooth muscle tissue is said to be arranged in a disorderly fashion because it is not striated like the other two types of muscle: cardiac and skeletal. Striations are lines that can only be seen with a microscope. *Smooth* muscle is typically found in the supporting tissues of hollow organs and blood vessels. *Cardiac* muscle is found exclusively in the heart; it is responsible for the contractions that pump blood throughout the body. *Skeletal* muscle, by far the most preponderant in the body, controls the movements of the skeleton. The contractions of skeletal muscle are responsible for all voluntary motion. There is no such thing as *rough* muscle.

30. C: *Melatonin* is produced by the pineal gland. One of the primary functions of melatonin is regulation of the circadian cycle, which is the rhythm of sleep and wakefulness. *Insulin* helps regulate the amount of glucose in the blood. Without insulin, the body is unable to convert blood sugar into energy. *Testosterone* is the main hormone produced by the testes; it is responsible for the development of adult male sex characteristics. *Epinephrine*, also known as adrenaline, performs a number of functions: It quickens and strengthens the heartbeat and dilates the bronchioles. Epinephrine is one of the hormones secreted when the body senses danger.

31. B: 0.05. In the metric system, 5 decimeters is equal to 0.05 decameters. A meter is the standard measurement of length. Prefixes are defined in increments of 10 to increase or decrease quantity.

- 139 -

The prefix "deci" is equivalent to 10-1 or a tenth (0.1). A decimeter would be equal to 0.1 meters. The prefix "deca" is equivalent to 10 or 101. A decameter would be equal to 10 meters. To convert a smaller unit to a larger one, move the decimal place to the left. Since 10 decimeters make up 1 meter, for 5 decimeters, move the decimal 1 place to the left to find meters, which would be 0.5 meters. Because a decameter is larger than 1 meter (10 meters in 1 decameter), move the decimal another place to the left to change from meters to decameters, which would be 0.05 decameters. An alternate method is to set up conversion factors. This method involves canceling units and is very helpful to learn for other scientific problems.

32. C: The distribution of weight among players of a football team. In this case, a pie chart can illustrate the whole number of players as well as the number (or percentage) of players at given weights. It would be easy to interpret the data that, for example, 75% of the team weigh 250 pounds or more, 20% weigh between 200 and 250 pounds, and a mere 5% weight less than 200 pounds. The other answers would be better served in bar or line charts to compare variables or amounts that do not vary greatly.

33. D: Electrophoresis. Electrophoresis, also known as gel electrophoresis, uses electrical charges to separate substances such as protein, DNA and RNA. Depending upon the electrical charge and size of the molecules, they will travel through a porous gel at different rates when a charge is applied. Answer A, Spectrophotometry, refers to the measurement of visible light, near-ultraviolet, and near-infrared wavelengths. Answer B, Chromatography, refers to a number of techniques that separate mixtures of chemicals based on the differences in the compound's affinity for a stationary phase, usually a porous solid, and a mobile phase, which can be either a liquid or a gas. Answer C, Centrifugation, separates mixtures by spinning to generate centripetal force, which causes heavier particles to separate from lighter particles.

34. A: By multiplying the ocular lens power times the objective being used. When using a light microscope, total magnification is determined by multiplying the ocular lens power times the objective being used. The ocular lens refers to the eyepiece, which has one magnification strength, typically 10x. The objective lens also has a magnification strength, often 4x, 10x, 40x or 100x. Using a 10x eyepiece with the 4x objective lens will give a magnification strength of 40x. Using a 10x eyepiece with the 100x objective lens will give a magnification strength of 1,000x. The shorter lens is the lesser magnification; the longer lens is the greater magnification.

35. C: Decaying specimens are never permitted but unknown specimens are sometimes permitted. When performing a dissection in class, decaying specimens can be permitted but unknown specimens are never permitted. Answer A, Rinse the specimen before handling, can help wash away excess preservative, which may be irritating. Answer B, Dispose of harmful chemicals according to district regulations; this is always required. Answer D, Students with open sores on their hands that cannot be covered should be excused from the dissection, is a good precaution. Exposure to pathogens and toxic chemicals can occur through open breaks in the skin.

36. A: Dispose of the solutions according to local disposal procedures. Solutions and compounds used in labs may be hazardous according to state and local regulatory agencies and should be treated with such precaution. Answer B, Empty the solutions into the sink and rinse with warm water and soap, does not take into account the hazards associated with a specific solution in terms of vapors, or interactions with water, soap and waste piping systems. Answer C, Ensure the solutions are secured in closed containers and throw away, may allow toxic chemicals to get into landfills and subsequently into fresh water systems. Answer D, Store the solutions in a secured, dry

place for later use, is incorrect as chemicals should not be re-used due to the possibility of contamination.

37. C: 20 g/L. One way to measure the density of an irregularly shaped object is to submerge it in water and measure the displacement. This is done by taking the mass (40 grams), then finding the volume by measuring how much water it displaces. Fill a graduated cylinder with water and record the amount. Put the object in the water and record the water level. Subtract the difference in water levels to get the amount of water displaced, which is also the volume of the object. In this case, 4.5 liters minus 2.5 liters equals 2 liters. Divide mass by volume (40 grams divided by 2 liters) to get 20 g/L (grams per liter).

38. B: A spoiling apple. A spoiling apple is an example of a chemical change. During a chemical change, one substance is changed into another. Oxidation, a chemical change, occurs when an apple spoils. Answer A, Sublimation of water, refers to the conversion between the solid and the gaseous phases of matter, with no intermediate liquid stage. This is a phase change, not a chemical reaction. Answer C, Dissolution of salt in water, refers to a physical change, since the salt and water can be separated again by evaporating the water, which is a physical change. Answer D, Pulverized rock, is an example of a physical change where the form has changed but not the substance itself.

39. D: The amount of potential energy an object has depends on mass, height above ground and gravitational attraction, but not temperature. The formula for potential energy is PE = mgh, or potential energy equals mass times gravity times height. Answers A, B, and C are all valid answers as they are all contained in the formula for potential energy. Potential energy is the amount of energy stored in a system particularly because of its position.

40. D: Elements on the periodic table are arranged into periods, or rows, according to atomic number, which is the number of protons in the nucleus. The periodic table illustrates the recurrence of properties. Each column, or group, contains elements that share similar properties, such as reactivity.

41. A: It takes half the amount of energy to increase the temperature of a 1 kg sample of ice by 1°C than a 1 kg sample of water. Heat capacity refers to the amount of heat or thermal energy required to raise the temperature of a specific substance a given unit. A substance with a higher heat capacity requires more heat to raise its temperature than a substance with a lower heat capacity. The comparison here is that the specific heat capacity of ice is half as much as that of liquid water, so it takes half the amount of energy to increase the same amount of ice one temperature unit than it would if it were liquid water.

42. D: Its temperature remains the same due to the latent heat of fusion. The temperature of a substance during the time of any phase change remains the same. In this case, the phase change was from liquid to solid, or freezing. Latent heat of fusion, in this case, is energy that is released from the substance as it reforms its solid form. This energy will be released and the liquid will turn to solid before the temperature of the substance will decrease further. If the substance were changing from solid to liquid, the heat of fusion would be the amount of heat required to break apart the attractions between the molecules in the solid form to change to the liquid form. The latent heat of fusion is exactly the same quantity of energy for a substance for either melting or freezing. Depending on the process, this amount of heat would either be absorbed by the substance (melting) or released (freezing).

43. B: A long nail or other type of metal, substance or matter that is heated at one end and then the other end becomes equally hot is an example of conduction. Conduction is energy transfer by neighboring molecules from an area of hotter temperature to cooler temperature. Answer A, Radiation, or thermal radiation, refers to heat being transferred through empty space by electromagnetic radiation. An example is sunlight heating the earth. Answer C, Convection, refers to heat being transferred by molecules moving from one location in the substance to another creating a heat current, usually in a gas or a liquid. Answer D, Entropy, relates to the second law of thermodynamics and refers to how much heat or energy is no longer available to do work in a system. It can also be stated as the amount of disorder in a system.

44. C: Heat transfer can never occur from a cooler object to a warmer object. While the second law of thermodynamics implies that heat never spontaneously transfers from a cooler object to a warmer object, it is possible for heat to be transferred to a warmer object, given the proper input of work to the system. This is the principle by which a refrigerator operates. Work is done to the system to transfer heat from the objects inside the refrigerator to the air surrounding the refrigerator. All other answer choices are true.

45. B: The measure of energy within a system is called heat. Answer A, temperature, is a measurement of the average kinetic energy of molecules in a substance. A higher temperature means greater kinetic energy or faster moving molecules. Answer C, entropy, is the amount of energy that is no longer available for work, related to the second law of thermodynamics. Answer D, thermodynamics, is the study of the conversion of energy into heat and work in a system.

46. D: It has a different number of neutrons than its element. An isotope is a variation of an element that has a different number of neutrons. The element and its various isotopes continue to have the same numbers of protons and electrons. For example, carbon has three naturally occurring isotopes, carbon-12, carbon-13 and carbon-14, which is radioactive. Isotopes of an element differ in mass number, which is the number of protons and neutrons added together, but have the same atomic number, or number of protons.

47. D: It is a stable atom. If an atom's outer shell is filled, it is a stable atom. The outer shell refers to one of many energy levels, or shells, that electrons occupy around a nucleus. An atom whose outer shell is not filled wants to become stable by filling the outer shell. It fills its outer shell by forming bonds. The atom can do this by gaining electrons or losing electrons in ionic compounds, or if the atom is a part of a molecule, by sharing electrons. If an atom has a full outer shell, such as the noble gases, it does not readily react with other atoms and does not exchange electrons to form bonds. These atoms are known as inert. Therefore, Answers A and B cannot be true. Answer C, It has 32 electrons in its outer shell, is not necessarily true because not all elements have the fourth shell that can hold 32 electrons. Some have fewer shells that hold fewer electrons.

48. A: Fission is a nuclear process where atomic nuclei split apart to form smaller nuclei. Nuclear fission can release large amounts of energy, emit gamma rays and form daughter products. It is used in nuclear power plants and bombs. Answer B, Fusion, refers to a nuclear process whereby atomic nuclei join to form a heavier nucleus, such as with stars. This can release or absorb energy depending upon the original elements. Answer C, Decay, refers to an atomic nucleus spontaneously losing energy and emitting ionizing particles and radiation. Answer D, Ionization, refers to a process by which atoms obtain a positive or negative charge because the number of electrons does not equal that of protons.

49. B: Electrons with greater amounts of energy are found farther from the nucleus than electrons with less energy. The principle quantum number describes the level or shell that an electron is in. The lower the number, the closer the electron is to the nucleus and the lower it is in energy.

50. D: The process whereby a radioactive element releases energy slowly over a long period of time to lower its energy and become more stable is best described as decay. The nucleus undergoing decay, known as the parent nuclide, spontaneously releases energy most commonly through the emission of an alpha particle, a beta particle or a gamma ray. The changed nucleus, called the daughter nuclide, is now more stable than the parent nuclide, although the daughter nuclide may undergo another decay to an even more stable nucleus. A decay chain is a series of decays of a radioactive element into different more stable elements.

51. C: A screw is a type of simple machine. A screw is an inclined plane wrapped around a shaft. A wedge is also an inclined plane. A compound machine is a machine that employs two or more simple machines. Answer A, a bicycle, is a compound machine, consisting of a combination of the simple machines: wheels, levers, pulleys and wedges (used as stoppers). Answer B, a pair of scissors, is also a compound machine consisting of two wedges (the blades) that pivot on a lever. Answer D, a shovel, is a compound machine consisting of a lever (the handle) and a wedge (the head of the shovel).

52. D: Mario balances a book on his head and walks across the room. In this example, work is not applied to the book by Mario. Work is defined as a force acting on an object to cause displacement. In this case, the book was not displaced in the direction of the force applied to it. Mario's head applied a vertical force to the book. By moving horizontally across the room, the movement of the book was not in the direction of the force applied. Therefore, there was no work applied to the book by Mario. In Answer A, Mario moves a book from the floor to the top shelf. Mario lifted the book vertically, in the same direction as the force applied. Therefore, work was done. In Answer B, A book drops off the shelf and falls to the floor, gravity has acted as the force and work was done. In Answer C, Mario pushes a box of books across the room, is also an example of work.

53. C: The ball will move forwards. Newton's first law of motion states that an object in motion tends to stay in motion until a force acts to change it. The ball is moving forward with the boat. When the front of the boat hits the dock, the ball's motion does not change. It continues to move forward because the force acting to stop the boat is not acting upon the ball. The forward motion of the boat is halted by the dock. The forward motion of the ball is not stopped. Since the ball is round there is little friction to provide an equal and opposite reaction to the forward motion.

54. A: Acceleration and centripetal force. Acceleration and centripetal force are required for circular motion to occur. Acceleration is defined as a change in direction of velocity. Centripetal force is toward the center, or inward force. Answer B, Acceleration and gravitational force, is incorrect because the force of gravity is not required for circular motion. Answer C, Constant speed and centripetal force, is also incorrect as constant speed is not required for circular motion to occur. Speed can vary and circular motion can still occur. Answer D, Constant speed and gravitational force is also incorrect as constant speed nor gravitational force are required for circular motion to occur.

55. B: Where the pipe is narrowest. A fluid, either a gas or a liquid, will flow faster through a narrow section of a pipe than a wider section of pipe. Bernoulli's Principle says that the faster a fluid flows, the less pressure the fluid exerts. Therefore, a fluid will exert a lower amount of pressure in the narrow section of pipe. A fluid moving through the pipe has the same flow throughout the wider

- 143 -

and narrow portions. This means that the same volume and mass of fluid must go a specific distance in a certain amount of time. In a narrow portion of pipe, there is less area for the same volume and mass of fluid to flow, so the fluid must move faster to maintain the same flow as in the wider portion of pipe. A fluid moving faster through a narrow portion of pipe will exert less pressure and a fluid moving slower through a wide section of pipe will exert a greater pressure.

56. A: The charge on the glass rod is positive and the charge on the cloth is negative when the glass rod is rubbed with a cloth made of polyester. This is an example of static electricity — the collection of electrically charged particles on the surface of a material. A static charge can be quickly discharged, commonly called a "spark", or discharged more slowly by dissipating to the ground. A static charge occurs because different materials have a capacity for giving up electrons and becoming positive (+), or for attracting electrons and becoming negative (-). The triboelectric series is a list of materials and their propensities for either giving up electrons to become positive or to gain the electrons to become negative. Polyester has a tendency to gain electrons to become negative and glass has a tendency to lose electrons to become positive.

57. B: Voltage and current are directly proportional to one another. Ohm's Law states that voltage and current in an electrical circuit are directly proportional to one another. Ohm's Law can be expressed as V=IR, where V is voltage, I is current and R is resistance. Voltage is also known as electrical potential difference and is the force that moves electrons through a circuit. For a given amount of resistance, an increase in voltage will result in an increase in current. Resistance and current are inversely proportional to each other. For a given voltage, an increase in resistance will result in a decrease in current.

58. C: In an atom with paired electrons, the opposite spins of each electron in the pair cancel out the magnetic field of each electron. A material becomes magnetic when the individual electrons of an atom spin unpaired thus allowing their magnetic fields to add together. The spin of an unpaired electron generates its own magnetic field. This can be used to make a magnet. When an external magnetic field is applied, these spins are lined up and the combined forces make a magnet.

59. D: Voltage is the same for each path and current is greatest in path C. In a parallel circuit, the voltage is the same for all three paths. Because the resistance is different on each path but the voltage is the same, Ohm's law dictates that the current will also be different for each path. Ohm's law says that current is inversely related to resistance. Therefore, the current will be greatest in path C as it has the least resistance, 2 ohms.

60. B: High temperature and humidity. Sound travels the farthest with high temperature and humidity. Sound is a mechanical wave. The sound wave travels through matter by causing a molecule to vibrate which then collides with a neighboring molecule causing it to vibrate and so on. A solid whose molecules are closely packed together will transmit the wave faster than a liquid or a gas whose particles are further apart. This is because the solid particles are more rigid and will respond to the disturbance quicker than a liquid or a gas, whose molecules are fluid. For this reason, solids can also propagate a wave further than a liquid or a gas. The principles of how sound travels through a solid can be applied to sound traveling through the air, as in this question. Air that is high in humidity has a higher density than dry air and can propagate the sound wave faster and farther than dry air. Sound waves also travel faster and farther at high temperatures. This is because at higher temperatures molecules have more kinetic energy to transmit the sound wave. At higher temperatures, molecules will also have more collisions which will result in the sound wave traveling farther and faster.

Special Report: Musculature/Innervation Review of the Arm and Back

Muscle	Origin	Insertion	Nerve
Trapezius	Ext. Occipit Protuberance, Spines of T Vertebrae	Lateral Clavicle, Spine of the Scapula	Spinal Accessory Nerve CN XI
Latissimus Dorsi	Spines of Lower 6 T Vertebrae, Iliac Crest and Lower 4 Ribs	Bicipital Groove	Thoracodorsal
Levator Scapulae	Transverse Process of C1-C4	Upper Medial Border of Scapula	Dorsal Scapula
Rhomboid Major	Spinous Process of T2-T5	Medial Border Scapula Below Spine	Dorsal Scapular
Rhomboid Minor	Spinous Process of C7-T1	Medial Border Scapula Opp. Spine	Dorsal Scapular
Teres Major	Lateral Dorsal Inferior Angle of Scapula	Bicipital Groove	Lower Subscapular
Teres Minor	Lateral Scapula 2/3 way down	Greater Tubercle of Humerus	Axillary
Deltoid	Lateral 1/3 Clavicle and Acromion Process, Spine of the Scapula	Deltoid Tuberosity	Axillary
Supraspinatus	Supraspinatus Fossa	Greater Tubercle of Humerus	Suprascapular
Infraspinatus	Infaspinatus Fossa	Greater Tubercle of Humerus	Suprascapular
Subscapularis	Subscapular Fossa	Lesser Tubercle of Humerus	Upper and lower Subscapular
Serratus Anterior	Slips of Upper 8-9 Ribs	Ventral-Medial Border Scapula	Long Thoracic
Subclavius	Inferior Surface of the Clavicle	First Rib	Nerve to the Subclavius
Pectoralis Major	Medial ½ clavicle and Side of Sternum	Bicipital Groove	Medial and Lateral Pectoral
Pectoralis Minor	Ribs 3,4,5 or 2,3,4	Coracoid Process	Medial Pectoral
Biceps Branchii	Supraglenoid Tubercle	Posterior Margin of Radial Tuberosity	Musculocutaneous
Coracobrachialis	Coracoid Process	Medial Humerus at Deltoid Tuberosity Level	Musculocutaneous
Brachialis	Anterior-Lateral ½ of Humerus	Ulnar Tuberosity and Coronoid Process	Musculocutaneous
Triceps Brachii	Infraglenoid Tubercle, Below and Medial to the Radial Groove	Olecranon Process	Radial
Anconeus	Posterior, Lateral Humeral Condyle	Upper Posterior Ulna	Radial
Brachioradialis	Lateral Supracondylar Ridge of Humerus	Radial Styloid Process	Radial
Pronator Teres	Medial Epicondyle and Supracondylar Ridge	½ Way Down on Lateral Radius	Median
Pronator Quadratus	Distal-Medial Ulna	Distal-Lateral Radius	Anterior Interosseous

Musculature/Innervation Review of the Forearm

Muscle	Origin	Insertion	Nerve
Brachioradialis	Lateral Supracondylar Ridge of Humerus	Radial Styloid Process	Radial
Pronator Teres	Medial Epicondyle and Supracondylar Ridge	½ Way Down on Lateral Radius	Median
Pronator Quadratus	Distal-Medial Ulna	Distal-Lateral Radius	Anterior Interosseous
Supinator	Lateral Epicondyle of Humerus	Upper ½ Lateral, Posterior Radius	Posterior Inter-Deep Radial
Flexor Carpi Radialis	Medial Epicondyle of Humerus	2nd and 3rd Metacarpal	Median
Flexor Carpi Ulnaris	Medial Epicondyle of Humerus	Pisiform, Hamate, 5th Metacarpal	Ulnar
Palmaris Longus	Medial Epicondyle of the Humerus	Palmar Aponeurosis and Flexor Retinaculum	Median
Flexor Digitorum Suerficialis	Medial Epicondyle, Radius, Ulna	Medial 4 Digits	Median
Flexor Digitorum Profundus	Ulna, Interosseous Membrane	Medial 4 Digits (distal part)	Median (lateral 2 digits), Ulnar (median 2 digits)
Flexor Pollicis Longus	Radius	Distal Phalanx (thumb)	Anterior Inter-Deep Median
Extensor Carpi Radialis Longus	Lateral Condyle and Supracondylar Ridge	2nd Metacarpal	Radial
Extensor Carpi Radialis Brevis	Lateral Epicondyle of Humerus	3rd Metacarpal	Posterior Inter-Deep Radial
Extensor Carpi Ulnaris	Lateral Epicondyle of Humerus	5th Metacarpal	Posterior Inter-Deep Radial
Extensor Digitorum	Lateral Epicondyle of Humerus	Extension Expansion Hood of Medial 4 Digits	Posterior Inter-Deep Radial
Extensor Digiti Minimi	Lateral Epicondyle of Humerus	Extension Expansion Hood of (little finger)	Posterior Inter-Deep Radial
Abductor Pollicis Longus	Posterior Radius and Ulna	Radial Side of 1st Metacarpal	Posterior Inter-Deep Radial
Extensor Indicis	Ulna and Interosseous Membrane	Extension Expansion Hood (index finger)	Posterior Inter-Deep Radial
Extensor Pollicis Longus	Ulna and Interosseous Membrane	Distal Phalanx (thumb)	Posterior Inter-Deep Radial
Extensor Pollicis Brevis	Radius	Proximal Phalanx (thumb)	Posterior Inter-Deep Radial

Musculature/Innervation Review of the Hand

Muscle	Origin	Insertion	Nerve
Adductor Policis	Capitate and Base of Adjacent Metacarpals	Proximal Phalanx (thumb)	Deep Branch of Ulnar
Lumbricals	Tendons of Flexor Digitorum Profundas	Extension Expansion Hood of Medial 4 Digits	Deep Branch Ulnar (medial 2 Ls), Median (lateral 2 Ls)
Dorsal Interosseous Muscles (4)	Sides of Metacarpals	Extension Expansion Hood of Digits 2-4	Deep Branch Ulnar
Palmar Interosseous (3)	Sides of Metacarpals	Extension Expansion Hood, Digits 2,4,5	Deep Branch Ulnar
Palmaris Brevis	Anterior Flexor Retinaculum and Palmar Aponeurosis	Skin-Ulnar Border of Hand	Superficial Ulnar
Abductor Pollicis Brevis	Flexor Retinaculum, Trapezium	Lateral Proximal Phalanx (thumb)	Median (thenar branch)
Flexor Pollicis Brevis	Flexor Retinaculum, Trapezium	Lateral Proximal Phalanx (thumb)	Median (thenar branch)
Opponens Pollicis	Flexor Retinaculum, Trapezium	Radial Border (1st Metacarpal)	Median (thenar branch)
Abductor Digiti Minimi	Flexor Retinaculum, Pisiform	Proximal Phalanx (little finger)	Deep Branch Ulnar
Flexor Digiti Minimi	Flexor Retinaculum, Hamate	Proximal Phalanx (little finger)	Deep Branch Ulnar
Opponens Digiti Minimi	Flexor Retinaculum, Hamate	Ulnar Medial Border (5th Metacarpal)	Deep Branch Ulnar

Musculature/Innervation Review of the Thigh

Muscle	Origin	Insertion	Nerve
Psoas Major	Bodies and Discs of T12-L5	Lesser Trochanter	L2,3
Psoas Minor	Bodies and Discs of T12 and L1	Pectineal Line of Superior Pubic Bone	L2,3
Iliacus	Upper 2/3 Iliac Fossa	Lesser Trochanter	Femoral L2-4
Pectinius	Pubic Ramus	Spiral Line	Femoral
Iliposoas	Joining of Psoas Major and Iliacus	Lesser Trochanter	L2-4
Piriformis	Anterior Surface of the Sacrum	Greater Trochanter	S1, S2
Obturator Internus	Inner Surface of the Obturator Membrane	Greater Trochanter	Sacral Plexus
Obturator Externus	Outer Surface of the Obturator Membrane	Greater Trochanter	Obturator
Gemellus Superior	Ischial Spine	Greater Trochanter	Sacral Plexus
Gemellus Inferior	Ischial Tuberosity	Greater Trochanter	Sacral Plexus
Quadratus Femoris	Ischial Tuberosity	Quadrate Tubercle of the Femur	Sacral Plexus
Gluteus Maximus	Outer Surface of Ilium, Sacrum and Coccyx	Iliotibial Tract, Gluteal Tubercle of the Femur	Inferior Gluteal
Gluteus Minimus	Outer Surface of the Ilium	Greater Trochanter	Superior Gluteal
Gluteus Medius	Outer Surface of the Ilium	Greater Trochanter	Superior Gluteal
Satorius	Anterior Superior Iliac Spine	Upper Medial Tibia	Femoral
Quadriceps Femoris	Anterior Inferior Iliac Spine, Femur-Lateral and Medial	Tibial Tuberosity	Femoral
Gracilis	Pubic Bone	Upper Medial Tibia	Obturator (anterior branch)
Abductor Longus	Pubic Bone	Linea Aspera	Obturator (anterior branch)
Abductor Brevis	Pubic Bone	Linea Aspera	Obturator (anterior branch)
Abductor Magnus	Pubic Bone	Entire Linea Aspera	Sciatic, Obturator
Tensor Faciae Latae	Iliac Crest	Iliotibial Band	Superior Gluteal
Biceps Femoris	Ischial Tuberosity, Linea Aspera	Head of Fibula, Lateral Condyle of Tibia	Sciatic-Tibial portion and Common Peroneal Portion
Semimembranosus	Ischial Tuberosity	Upper Medial Tibia	Sciatic-Tibial Portion
Semitendinosus	Ischial Tuberosity	Upper Medial Tibia	Sciatic-Tibial Portion

Musculature/Innervation Review of the Calf and Foot

Muscle	Origin	Insertion	Nerve
Tibialis Anterior	Upper 2/3 Lateral Tibia and Interosseous Membrane	1st Cuneiform and Base of 1st Metatarsal	Deep Peroneal
Extensor Digitorum Longus	Upper 2/3 Fibula and Interosseous Membrane	4 Tendons-Distal Middle Phalanges	Deep Peroneal
Extensor Hallucis Longus	Middle 1/3 of Anterior Fibula	Base of Distal Phalanx of Big Toe	Deep Peroneal
Peroneus Tertius	Distal Fibula	Base of 5th Metatarsal	Deep Peroneal
Extensor Hallucis Brevis	Dorsal Calcaneus	Extensor Digitorum Longus Tendons	Deep Peroneal
Peroneus Longus	Upper 2/3 Lateral Fibula	1st Metatarsal and 1st Cuneiform	Superficial Peroneal
Peroneus Brevis	Lateral Distal Fibula	5th Metatarsal Tuberosity	Superficial Peroneal
Soleus	Upper Shaft of Fibula	Calcaneus via Achilles Tendon	Tibial
Flexor Digitorum Longus	Middle 1/3 of Posterior Tibia	Base of Distal Phalanx of Lateral 4 Toes	Tibial
Flexor Hallucis Longus	Middle and Lower 1/3 of Posterior Tibia	Distal Phalanx of Big Toe	Tibial
Tibialis Posterior	Posterior Upper Tibia, Fibula	Navicular Bone and 1st Cuneiform	Tibial
Popliteus	Upper Posterior Tibia	Lateral Condyle of Femur	Tibial
Flexor Digitorum Brevis	Calcaneus	Middle Phalanges of Lateral 4 Toes	Medial Plantar
Abductor Hallucis	Calcaneus	Medial Proximal Phalanx of Big Toe	Medial Plantar
Abductor Digiti Brevis	Calcaneus	Lateral Proximal Phalanx of Big Toe	Lateral Plantar
Quadratus Plantae	Lateral and Medial Side of the Calcaneus	Tendons of Flexor Digitorum Longus	Lateral Plantar
Lumbricals	Tendons of Flexor Digitorum Longus	Extensor Tendons of Toes	Medial Plantar/Lateral Plantar
Flexor Hallucis Brevis	Cuboid Bone	Splits on Base of Proximal Phalanx of Big Toe	Medial Plantar
Flexor Digiti Minimi Brevis	Base of 5th Metatarsal	Base of Proximal Phalanx of Little Toe	Lateral Plantar
Abductor Hallucis	Metatarsals 2-4	Base of Proximal Phalanx of Big Toe	Lateral Plantar
Interossei	Sides of Metatarsal Bones	Base of 1st Phalanx and Extensor Tendons	Lateral Plantar

CPR Guidelines for Professional Rescuers

Topic	Adult	Child	Infant
	Past puberty	1 y/o - puberty	Under 1 y/o
Conscious Choking	abdominal thrusts (or chest thrusts in pregnant/obese)	abdominal thrusts	5 back slaps and 5 chest thrusts in infant
Unconscious Choking	Begin chest compression. Look in the victim's mouth for foreign body before giving breaths.		
Rescue Breaths Normal breath given over 1 second until chest rises.	10-12 breaths per minute (1 breath every 6-8 seconds)	12-20 breaths per minute (1 breath every 3-5 seconds)	20 breaths per minute (1 breath every 3 seconds)
Chest Compressions to Ventilation Ratios (Single Rescuer)	30:2		
Chest Compressions to Ventilation Ratios (Two Rescuer)	30:2	15:2	
Chest Compression rate	At least 100/minute		
Chest Compression Land Marking Method	two hands center of the chest, even with nipples	one hand center of the chest even with nipples	2 or 3 fingers, just below the nipple line at the center of the chest
Chest Compression Depth	At least 2" compression (hands overlapping)	about 2" compression or 1/3 the AP diameter (only heel of one hand)	about 1 ½" compression or 1/3 the AP diameter (2 fingers)
Activate Emergency Response System	As soon as you realize that the victim is unresponsive	After 5 cycles of CPR	After 5 cycles of CPR

Checklist:
- Check the scene
- Check for responsiveness – ask, "Are you OK?"
- Adult - call 911, <u>then</u> administer CPR
- Child/Infant – administer CPR for 5 cycles, <u>then</u> call 911
- Open victim's airway and check for breathing
- Two rescue breaths should be given, 1 second each, and should produce a visible chest rise
- If the air does not go in, reposition and try 2 breaths again
- Check victim's pulse – chest compressions are recommended if an infant or child has a rate less than 60 per minute with signs of poor perfusion
- Continue 30:2 ratio until victim moves, AED is brought to the scene, or professional help arrives

Special Report: Pharmacology Generic/Trade Names of 50+ Key Drugs in Medicine

Brand Name	Generic
Synthroid	Levothyroxine
Crestor	Rosuvastatin
Ventolin	Albuterol
Nexium	Esomeprazole
Advair	Fluticasone / Salmeterol
Lantus	Insulin glargine
Vyvanse	Lisdexamfetamine
Lyrica	Pregabalin
Spiriva	Tiotropium
Januvia	Sitagliptin
Abilify	Aripiprazole
Symbicort	Budesonide / Formoterol
Tamiflu	Oseltamivir
Cialis	Tadalafil
Viagra	Sildenafil
Suboxone	Buprenorphine
Zetia	Ezetimibe
Xarelto	Rivaroxaban
Bystolic	Nebivolol
Celebrex	Celecoxib
Nasonex	Mometasone furoate
Namenda	Memantine
Flovent	Fluticasone
Oxycontin	Oxycodone
Diovan	Valsartan
Voltaren	Diclofenac
Dexilant	Dexlansoprazole
Benicar	Olmesartan
Vesicare	Solifenacin
Lumigan	Bimatoprost
Pataday	Olopatadine
Travatan	Travoprost
Toprol-XL	Metoprolol
Pristiq	Desvenlafaxine
Invokana	Canagliflozin
Strattera	Atomoxetine

Seroquel	Quetiapine
Focalin	Dexmethylphenidate
Victoza	Liraglutide
Exelon	Rivastigmine
Tradjenta	Linagliptin
Enbrel	Etanercept
Onglyza	Saxagliptin
Ranexa	Ranolazine
Truvada	Emtricitabine / Tenofovir
Welchol	Colesevelam
Linzess	Linaclotide
Latuda	Lurasidone
Alphagan	Brimonidine
Viibryd	Vilazodone
Effient	Prasugrel
Norvir	Ritonavir
Amitiza	Lubiprostone
Uloric	Febuxostat
Lotemax	Loteprednol

Special Report: Difficult Patients

Every professional will eventually get a difficult patient on their list of responsibilities. These patients can be mentally, physically, and emotionally combative in many different environments. Consequently, care of these patients should be conducted in a manner for personal and self-protection of the professional. Some of the key guidelines are as follows:

1. Never allow yourself to be cornered in a room with the patient positioned between you and the door.
2. Don't escalate the tension with verbal bantering. Basically, don't argue with the patient or resident.
3. Ask permission before performing any normal tasks in a patient's room whenever possible.
4. Discuss your concerns with nursing staff. Consult the floor supervisor if necessary, especially when safety is an issue.
5. Get help from other support staff when offering care. Get a witness if you are anticipating abuse of any kind.
6. Remove yourself from the situation if you are concerned about your personal safety at all times.
7. If attacked, defend yourself with the force necessary for self-protection and attempt to separate from the patient.
8. Be aware of the patient's medical and mental history prior to entering the patient's room.
9. Don't put yourself in a position to be hurt.
10. Get the necessary help for all transfers, bathing and dressing activities from other staff members for difficult patients.
11. Respect the resident and patient's personal property.
12. Get assistance quickly, via the call bell or vocal projection, if a situation becomes violent or abuse.
13. Immediately seek medical treatment if injured.
14. Fill out an incident report for proper documentation of the occurrence.
15. Protect other patients from abusive behavior.

Special Report: Guidelines for Standard Precautions

Standard precautions are precautions taken to avoid contracting various diseases and preventing the spread of disease to those who have compromised immunity. Some of these diseases include human immunodeficiency virus (HIV), acquired immunodeficiency syndrome (AIDS), and hepatitis B (HBV). Standard precautions are needed since many diseases do not display signs or symptoms in their early stages. Standard precautions mean to treat all body fluids/ substances as if they were contaminated. These body fluids include but are not limited to the following blood, semen, vaginal secretions, breast milk, amniotic fluid, feces, urine, peritoneal fluid, synovial fluid, cerebrospinal fluid, secretions from the nasal and oral cavities, and lacrimal and sweat gland excretions. This means that standard precautions should be used with all patients.

1. A shield for the eyes and face must be used if there is a possibility of splashes from blood and body fluids.
2. If possibility of blood or body fluids being splashed on clothing, you must wear a plastic apron.
3. Gloves must be worn if you could possibly come in contact with blood or body fluids. They are also needed if you are going to touch something that may have come in contact with blood or body fluids.
4. Hands must be washed even if you were wearing gloves. Hands must be washed and gloves must be changed between patients. Wash hands with at a dime size amount of soap and warm water for about 30 seconds. Singing "Mary had a little lamb" is approximately 30 seconds.
5. Blood and body fluid spills must be cleansed and disinfected using a solution of one part bleach to 10 parts water or your hospitals accepted method.
6. Used needles must be separated from clean needles. Throw both the needle and the syringe away in the sharps' container. The sharps' container is mad of puncture proof material.
7. Take extra care in performing high-risk activities that include puncturing the skin and cutting the skin.
8. CPR equipment to be used in a hospital must include resuscitation bags and mouthpieces.

Special precautions must be taken to dispose of biomedical waste. Biomedical waste includes but is not limited to the following laboratory waste, pathology waste, liquid waste from suction, all sharp object, bladder catheters, chest tubes, IV tubes, and drainage containers. Biomedical waste is removed from a facility by trained biomedical waste disposers.

The health care professional is legally and ethically responsible for adhering to standard precautions. They may prevent you from contracting a fatal disease or from a patient contracting a disease from you that could be deadly.

Special Report: Basic Review of Types of Fractures

A fracture is defined as a break in a bone that may sometimes involve cartilaginous structures. A fracture can be classified according to its cause or the type of break. The following definitions are used to describe breaks.

1. Traumatic fracture – break in a bone resulting from injury
2. Spontaneous fracture – break in a bone resulting from disease
3. Pathologic fracture – another name for a spontaneous fracture
4. Compound fracture – occurs when fracture bone is exposed to the outside by an opening in the skin
5. Simple fracture - occurs when a break is contained within the skin
6. Greenstick fracture - a traumatic break that is incomplete and occurs on the convex surface of the bend in the bone
7. Fissured fracture – a traumatic break that involves an incomplete longitudinal break
8. Comminuted fracture – a traumatic break that involves a complete fracture that results in several bony fragments
9. Transverse fracture – a traumatic break that is complete and occurs at a right angle to the axis of the bone
10. Oblique fracture- a traumatic break that occurs at an angle other than a right angle to the axis of the bone.
11. Spiral fracture – a traumatic break that occurs by twisting a bone with extreme force

A compound fracture is much more dangerous than a simple break. This is due to the break in skin that can allow microorganisms to infect the injured tissue. When a fracture occurs, blood vessels within the bone and its periosteum are disrupted. The periosteum, covering of fibrous connective tissue on the surface of the bone, may also be damaged or torn.

Secret Key #1 – Time is Your Greatest Enemy

To succeed, you must ration your time properly. The reason that time is so critical is that every question counts the same toward your final score. If you run out of time on any section, the questions that you do not answer will hurt your score far more than earlier questions that you spent extra time on and feel certain are correct.

Success Strategy #1

Pace Yourself

Wear a watch to the exam. At the beginning of the test, check the time (or start a chronometer on your watch to count the minutes), and check the time after each passage or every few questions to make sure you are "on schedule."

If you find that you are falling behind time during the test, you must speed up. Even though a rushed answer is more likely to be incorrect, it is better to miss a couple of questions by being rushed, than to completely miss later questions by not having enough time. It is better to end with more time than you need than to run out of time.

If you are forced to speed up, do it efficiently. Usually one or more answer choices can be eliminated without too much difficulty. Above all, don't panic. Don't speed up and just begin guessing at random choices. By pacing yourself, and continually monitoring your progress against your watch, you will always know exactly how far ahead or behind you are with your available time. If you find that you are a few minutes behind on a section, don't skip questions without spending any time on it, just to catch back up. Begin spending a little less time per question and after a few questions, you will have caught back up more gradually. Once you catch back up, you can continue working each problem at your normal pace. If you have time at the end, go back then and finish the questions that you left behind.

Furthermore, don't dwell on the problems that you were rushed on. If a problem was taking up too much time and you made a hurried guess, it must have been difficult. The difficult questions are the ones you are most likely to miss anyway, so it isn't a big loss.

Last minute guessing will be covered in the next chapter.

Lastly, sometimes it is beneficial to slow down if you are constantly getting ahead of time. You are always more likely to catch a careless mistake by working more slowly than quickly, and among very high-scoring students (those who are likely to have lots of time left over), careless errors affect the score more than mastery of material.

Scanning

Don't waste time reading, enjoying, and completely understanding the passage. Simply scan the passage to get a rough idea of what it is about. You will return to the passage for each question, so there is no need to memorize it. Only spend as much time scanning as is necessary to get a vague impression of its overall subject content.

Secret Key #2 – Guessing is not guesswork.

Most students do not understand the impact that proper guessing can have on their score. Unless you score extremely high, guessing will contribute a significant amount of points to your score.

Monkeys Take the Exam

What most students don't realize is that to insure that random 25% chance, you have to guess randomly. If you put 20 monkeys in a room to take the exam, assuming they answered once per question and behaved themselves, on average they would get 25% of the questions correct. Put 20 students in the room, and the average will be much lower among guessed questions. Why?

1. The exam intentionally has deceptive answer choices that "look" right. A student has no idea about a question, so picks the "best looking" answer, which is often wrong. The monkey has no idea what looks good and what doesn't, so will consistently be lucky about 25% of the time.
2. Students will eliminate answer choices from the guessing pool based on a hunch or intuition. Simple but correct answers often get excluded, leaving a 0% chance of being correct. The monkey has no clue, and often gets lucky with the best choice.

This is why the process of elimination endorsed by most test courses is flawed and detrimental to your performance- students don't guess, they make an ignorant stab in the dark that is usually worse than random.

Success Strategy #2

Let me introduce one of the most valuable ideas of this course- the $5 challenge:

You only mark your "best guess" if you are willing to bet $5 on it.
You only eliminate choices from guessing if you are willing to bet $5 on it.

Why $5? Five dollars is an amount of money that is small yet not insignificant, and can really add up fast (20 questions could cost you $100). Likewise, each answer choice on one question of the exam will have a small impact on your overall score, but it can really add up to a lot of points in the end.

The process of elimination IS valuable. The following shows your chance of guessing it right:

If you eliminate this many choices:	0	1	2	3
Chance of getting it correct	25%	33%	50%	100%

However, if you accidentally eliminate the right answer or go on a hunch for an incorrect answer, your chances drop dramatically: to 0%. By guessing among all the answer choices, you are GUARANTEED to have a shot at the right answer.

That's why the $5 test is so valuable- if you give up the advantage and safety of a pure guess, it had better be worth the risk.

What we still haven't covered is how to be sure that whatever guess you make is truly random. Here's the easiest way:

Always pick the first answer choice among those remaining.

Such a technique means that you have decided, **before you see a single test question**, exactly how you are going to guess- and since the order of choices tells you nothing about which one is correct, this guessing technique is perfectly random.

Specific Guessing Techniques

Similar Answer Choices

When you have two answer choices that are direct opposites, one of them is usually the correct answer.
Example:
  a. forward
  b. backward

These two answer choices are very similar and fall into the same family of answer choices. A family of answer choices is when two or three answer choices are very similar. Often two will be opposites and one may show an equality.
Example:
  a. excited
  b. overjoyed
  c. thrilled
  d. upset

Note how the first three choices are all related. They all ask describe a state of happiness. However, choice D is not in the same family of questions. Being upset is the direct opposite of happiness.

Summary of Guessing Techniques

1. Eliminate as many choices as you can by using the $5 test. Use the common guessing strategies to help in the elimination process, but only eliminate choices that pass the $5 test.
2. Among the remaining choices, only pick your "best guess" if it passes the $5 test.
3. Otherwise, guess randomly by picking the first remaining choice that was not eliminated.

Secret Key #3 – Practice Smarter, Not Harder

Many students delay the test preparation process because they dread the awful amounts of practice time they think necessary to succeed on the test. We have refined an effective method that will take you only a fraction of the time.

There are a number of "obstacles" in your way on the exam. Among these are answering questions, finishing in time, and mastering test-taking strategies. All must be executed on the day of the test at peak performance, or your score will suffer. The exam is a mental marathon that has a large impact on your future.

Just like a marathon runner, it is important to work your way up to the full challenge. So first you just worry about questions, and then time, and finally strategy:

Success Strategy #3

1. Find a good source for exam practice tests.
2. If you are willing to make a larger time investment (or if you want to really "learn" the material, a time consuming but ultimately valuable endeavor), consider buying one of the better study guides on the market
3. Take a practice test with no time constraints, with all study helps "open book." Take your time with questions and focus on applying the strategies.
4. Take another test, this time with time constraints, with all study helps "open book."
5. Take a final practice test with no open material and time limits.

If you have time to take more practice tests, just repeat step 5. By gradually exposing yourself to the full rigors of the test environment, you will condition your mind to the stress of test day and maximize your success.

Secret Key #4 – Prepare, Don't Procrastinate

Let me state an obvious fact: if you take the exam three times, you will get three different scores. This is due to the way you feel on test day, the level of preparedness you have, and, despite exam's claims to the contrary, some tests WILL be easier for you than others.

Since your acceptance will largely depend on your score, you should maximize your chances of success. In order to maximize the likelihood of success, you've got to prepare in advance. This means taking practice tests and spending time learning the information and test taking strategies you will need to succeed.

Since you have to pay a registration fee each time you take the exam, don't take it as a "practice" test. Feel free to take sample tests on your own, but when you go to take the exam, be prepared, be focused, and do your best the first time!

Secret Key #5 – Test Yourself

Everyone knows that time is money. There is no need to spend too much of your time or too little of your time preparing for the exam. You should only spend as much of your precious time preparing as is necessary for you to pass it.

Once you have taken a practice test under real conditions of time constraints, then you will know if you are ready for the test or not.

If you have scored extremely high the first time that you take the practice test, then there is not much point in spending countless hours studying. You are already there.

Benchmark your abilities by retaking practice tests and seeing how much you have improved. Once you score high enough to get accepted into the school of your choice, then you are ready.

If you have scored well below where you need, then knuckle down and begin studying in earnest. Check your improvement regularly through the use of practice tests under real conditions. Above all, don't worry, panic, or give up. The key is perseverance!

Then, when you go to take the exam, remain confident and remember how well you did on the practice tests. If you can score high enough on a practice test, then you can do the same on the real thing.

General Strategies

The most important thing you can do is to ignore your fears and jump into the test immediately- do not be overwhelmed by any strange-sounding terms. You have to jump into the test like jumping into a pool- all at once is the easiest way.

Make Predictions

As you read and understand the question, try to guess what the answer will be. Remember that several of the answer choices are wrong, and once you begin reading them, your mind will immediately become cluttered with answer choices designed to throw you off. Your mind is typically the most focused immediately after you have read the question and digested its contents. If you can, try to predict what the correct answer will be. You may be surprised at what you can predict. Quickly scan the choices and see if your prediction is in the listed answer choices. If it is, then you can be quite confident that you have the right answer. It still won't hurt to check the other answer choices, but most of the time, you've got it!

Answer the Question

It may seem obvious to only pick answer choices that answer the question, but the test writers can create some excellent answer choices that are wrong. Don't pick an answer just because it sounds right, or you believe it to be true. It MUST answer the question. Once you've made your selection, always go back and check it against the question and make sure that you didn't misread the question, and the answer choice does answer the question posed.

Benchmark

After you read the first answer choice, decide if you think it sounds correct or not. If it doesn't, move on to the next answer choice. If it does, mentally mark that answer choice. This doesn't mean that you've definitely selected it as your answer choice, it just means that it's the best you've seen thus far. Go ahead and read the next choice. If the next choice is worse than the one you've already selected, keep going to the next answer choice. If the next choice is better than the choice you've already selected, mentally mark the new answer choice as your best guess.

The first answer choice that you select becomes your standard. Every other answer choice must be benchmarked against that standard. That choice is correct until proven otherwise by another answer choice beating it out. Once you've decided that no other answer choice seems as good, do one final check to ensure that your answer choice answers the question posed.

Valid Information

Don't discount any of the information provided in the question. Every piece of information may be necessary to determine the correct answer. None of the information in the question is there to throw you off (while the answer choices will certainly have information to throw you off). If two seemingly unrelated topics are discussed, don't ignore either. You can be confident there is a relationship, or it wouldn't be included in the question, and you are probably going to have to determine what is that relationship to find the answer.

Avoid "Fact Traps"

Don't get distracted by a choice that is factually true. Your search is for the answer that answers the question. Stay focused and don't fall for an answer that is true but incorrect. Always go back to the question and make sure you're choosing an answer that actually answers the question and is not just a true statement. An answer can be factually correct, but it MUST answer the question asked. Additionally, two answers can both be seemingly correct, so be sure to read all of the answer choices, and make sure that you get the one that BEST answers the question.

Milk the Question

Some of the questions may throw you completely off. They might deal with a subject you have not been exposed to, or one that you haven't reviewed in years. While your lack of knowledge about the subject will be a hindrance, the question itself can give you many clues that will help you find the correct answer. Read the question carefully and look for clues. Watch particularly for adjectives and nouns describing difficult terms or words that you don't recognize. Regardless of if you completely understand a word or not, replacing it with a synonym either provided or one you more familiar with may help you to understand what the questions are asking. Rather than wracking your mind about specific detailed information concerning a difficult term or word, try to use mental substitutes that are easier to understand.

The Trap of Familiarity

Don't just choose a word because you recognize it. On difficult questions, you may not recognize a number of words in the answer choices. The test writers don't put "make-believe" words on the test; so don't think that just because you only recognize all the words in one answer choice means that answer choice must be correct. If you only recognize words in one answer choice, then focus on that one. Is it correct? Try your best to determine if it is correct. If it is, that is great, but if it doesn't, eliminate it. Each word and answer choice you eliminate increases your chances of getting the question correct, even if you then have to guess among the unfamiliar choices.

Eliminate Answers

Eliminate choices as soon as you realize they are wrong. But be careful! Make sure you consider all of the possible answer choices. Just because one appears right, doesn't mean that the next one won't be even better! The test writers will usually put more than one good answer choice for every question, so read all of them. Don't worry if you are stuck between two that seem right. By getting down to just two remaining possible choices, your odds are now 50/50. Rather than wasting too much time, play the odds. You are guessing, but guessing wisely, because you've been able to knock out some of the answer choices that you know are wrong. If you are eliminating choices and realize that the last answer choice you are left with is also obviously wrong, don't panic. Start over and consider each choice again. There may easily be something that you missed the first time and will realize on the second pass.

Tough Questions

If you are stumped on a problem or it appears too hard or too difficult, don't waste time. Move on! Remember though, if you can quickly check for obviously incorrect answer choices, your chances of guessing correctly are greatly improved. Before you completely give up, at least try to knock out a couple of possible answers. Eliminate what you can and then guess at the remaining answer choices before moving on.

Brainstorm

If you get stuck on a difficult question, spend a few seconds quickly brainstorming. Run through the complete list of possible answer choices. Look at each choice and ask yourself, "Could this answer the question satisfactorily?" Go through each answer choice and consider it independently of the other. By systematically going through all possibilities, you may find something that you would otherwise overlook. Remember that when you get stuck, it's important to try to keep moving.

Read Carefully

Understand the problem. Read the question and answer choices carefully. Don't miss the question because you misread the terms. You have plenty of time to read each question thoroughly and make sure you understand what is being asked. Yet a happy medium must be attained, so don't waste too much time. You must read carefully, but efficiently.

Face Value

When in doubt, use common sense. Always accept the situation in the problem at face value. Don't read too much into it. These problems will not require you to make huge leaps of logic. The test writers aren't trying to throw you off with a cheap trick. If you have to go beyond creativity and make a leap of logic in order to have an answer choice answer the question, then you should look at the other answer choices. Don't overcomplicate the problem by creating theoretical relationships or explanations that will warp time or space. These are normal problems rooted in reality. It's just that the applicable relationship or explanation may not be readily apparent and you have to figure things out. Use your common sense to interpret anything that isn't clear.

Prefixes

If you're having trouble with a word in the question or answer choices, try dissecting it. Take advantage of every clue that the word might include. Prefixes and suffixes can be a huge help. Usually they allow you to determine a basic meaning. Pre- means before, post- means after, pro - is positive, de- is negative. From these prefixes and suffixes, you can get an idea of the general meaning of the word and try to put it into context. Beware though of any traps. Just because con is the opposite of pro, doesn't necessarily mean congress is the opposite of progress!

Hedge Phrases

Watch out for critical "hedge" phrases, such as likely, may, can, will often, sometimes, often, almost, mostly, usually, generally, rarely, sometimes. Question writers insert these hedge phrases to cover every possibility. Often an answer choice will be wrong simply because it leaves no room for exception. Avoid answer choices that have definitive words like "exactly," and "always".

Switchback Words

Stay alert for "switchbacks". These are the words and phrases frequently used to alert you to shifts in thought. The most common switchback word is "but". Others include although, however, nevertheless, on the other hand, even though, while, in spite of, despite, regardless of.

New Information

Correct answer choices will rarely have completely new information included. Answer choices typically are straightforward reflections of the material asked about and will directly relate to the question. If a new piece of information is included in an answer choice that doesn't even seem to relate to the topic being asked about, then that answer choice is likely incorrect. All of the information needed to answer the question is usually provided for you, and so you should not have to make guesses that are unsupported or choose answer choices that require unknown information that cannot be reasoned on its own.

Time Management

On technical questions, don't get lost on the technical terms. Don't spend too much time on any one question. If you don't know what a term means, then since you don't have a dictionary, odds are you aren't going to get much further. You should immediately recognize terms as whether or not you know them. If you don't, work with the other clues that you have, the other answer choices and terms provided, but don't waste too much time trying to figure out a difficult term.

Contextual Clues

Look for contextual clues. An answer can be right but not correct. The contextual clues will help you find the answer that is most right and is correct. Understand the context in which a phrase or statement is made. This will help you make important distinctions.

Don't Panic

Panicking will not answer any questions for you. Therefore, it isn't helpful. When you first see the question, if your mind goes blank, take a deep breath. Force yourself to mechanically go through the steps of solving the problem and using the strategies you've learned.

Pace Yourself

Don't get clock fever. It's easy to be overwhelmed when you're looking at a page full of questions, your mind is full of random thoughts and feeling confused, and the clock is ticking down faster than you would like. Calm down and maintain the pace that you have set for yourself. As long as you are on track by monitoring your pace, you are guaranteed to have enough time for yourself. When you get to the last few minutes of the test, it may seem like you won't have enough time left, but if you only have as many questions as you should have left at that point, then you're right on track!

Answer Selection

The best way to pick an answer choice is to eliminate all of those that are wrong, until only one is left and confirm that is the correct answer. Sometimes though, an answer choice may immediately look right. Be careful! Take a second to make sure that the other choices are not equally obvious. Don't make a hasty mistake. There are only two times that you should stop before checking other answers. First is when you are positive that the answer choice you have selected is correct. Second is when time is almost out and you have to make a quick guess!

Check Your Work

Since you will probably not know every term listed and the answer to every question, it is important that you get credit for the ones that you do know. Don't miss any questions through careless mistakes. If at all possible, try to take a second to look back over your answer selection and make sure you've selected the correct answer choice and haven't made a costly careless mistake (such as marking an answer choice that you didn't mean to mark). This quick double check should more than pay for itself in caught mistakes for the time it costs.

Beware of Directly Quoted Answers

Sometimes an answer choice will repeat word for word a portion of the question or reference section. However, beware of such exact duplication – it may be a trap! More than likely, the correct choice will paraphrase or summarize a point, rather than being exactly the same wording.

Slang

Scientific sounding answers are better than slang ones. An answer choice that begins "To compare the outcomes…" is much more likely to be correct than one that begins "Because some people insisted…"

Extreme Statements

Avoid wild answers that throw out highly controversial ideas that are proclaimed as established fact. An answer choice that states the "process should be used in certain situations, if…" is much more likely to be correct than one that states the "process should be discontinued completely." The first is a calm rational statement and doesn't even make a definitive, uncompromising stance, using a hedge word "if" to provide wiggle room, whereas the second choice is a radical idea and far more extreme.

Answer Choice Families

When you have two or more answer choices that are direct opposites or parallels, one of them is usually the correct answer. For instance, if one answer choice states "x increases" and another answer choice states "x decreases" or "y increases," then those two or three answer choices are very similar in construction and fall into the same family of answer choices. A family of answer choices is when two or three answer choices are very similar in construction, and yet often have a directly opposite meaning. Usually the correct answer choice will be in that family of answer choices. The "odd man out" or answer choice that doesn't seem to fit the parallel construction of the other answer choices is more likely to be incorrect.

Additional Bonus Material

Due to our efforts to try to keep this book to a manageable length, we've created a link that will give you access to all of your additional bonus material.

Please visit http://www.mometrix.com/bonus948/psbrn to access the information.